Sarah Dickens

25

£3-75

CAT DOCTOR

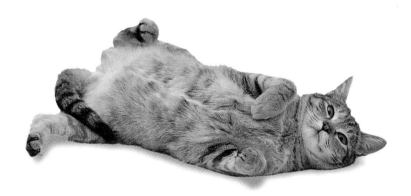

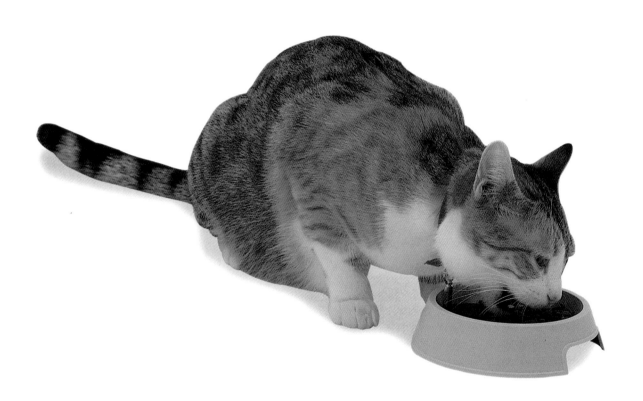

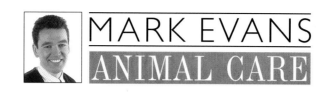

MARK EVANS
ANIMAL CARE

CAT DOCTOR

MITCHELL BEAZLEY

To Grandma, Andrew, Karen, 'Emma' and 'Sparky'

Executive Art Editor: Vivienne Brar
Commissioning Editor: Samantha Ward-Dutton
Project Editor: Jane Royston
Designer: Norma Martin
Production: Kate Thomas

First published in Great Britain in 1996 by Mitchell Beazley,
an imprint of Reed Consumer Books Limited,
Michelin House, 81 Fulham Road, London SW3 6RB and
Auckland, Melbourne, Singapore and Toronto

ISBN 1-85732-797-7

A CIP catalogue of this book is available at the British Library.

Printed in China

Sarah Dickens

Contents

Introduction

Contrary to popular belief, cats do not have 'nine lives'. Just like us mere mortals, they only have one. Having said this, it is true that some cats do appear to have an uncanny knack of recovering from serious injuries, often against all the odds. You would be as amazed as I always am – and owners certainly are – when as a result of nothing more than good nursing care a cat suddenly begins to walk again, having been paralysed since being injured in a road accident many weeks previously.

However, apparently 'miraculous' recoveries such as these should not fool you into believing that your cat will be equally fortunate should he be injured or become ill. All cats are vulnerable to a very large number of medical conditions – some extremely serious, others less so – and, when they are unwell, they suffer as we do.

Your cat's health

Caring for your cat's health and welfare is a team responsibility and, together with the staff at your vet centre, you are an essential part of that team. Through feeding your cat a good diet, ensuring that he has appropriate mental and physical exercise, and keeping up to date with his routine healthcare procedures such as grooming, parasite control and vaccination, you will help to keep him fit and well. However, despite your best efforts to do this, it is extremely likely that sooner or later he will suffer from accidental injury or illness. After all, it is a rare individual indeed – either human or feline – who manages to go through a lifetime with no medical problems of any kind.

When your cat is unwell in any way, he will rely on you to identify that there is something wrong with him, and to take prompt action to help him. Although a vet will be the only person who is suitably qualified to diagnose the full extent and cause of your cat's symptoms, and to instigate any appropriate treatment regime for him, you will be the only person able to offer your vet essential information concerning the history of your cat's illness or injury.

Cats are often extremely good at concealing the fact that they are unwell, so you should monitor your cat's behaviour closely and carry out regular and frequent health-checks in order to identify the earliest – often vague – symptoms associated with many conditions. It is very likely that you will also play a crucial role in nursing your cat through his recovery.

Seeking veterinary help

Make no mistake, this book is certainly not intended to encourage you to avoid seeking advice and expert assistance from your vet centre when your cat is either injured or ill. Believe me, there can be nothing more dangerous to a cat's welfare than an owner who, armed with only half the facts, refuses to recognize the limitations of his or her own knowledge about cat health and, as a result, fails to obtain professional veterinary care for his or her pet when it is needed.

For your cat's sake, you must be prepared to talk to a member of the staff at your vet centre promptly whenever you are concerned about your cat's health, no matter how trivial you think the problem may be. However, try not to pester your vet with general questions on caring for your cat. Many good vet centres employ one or more highly trained veterinary nurses, who should be happy to provide you with expert general advice on any health, behavioural or cat-care matters, either over the telephone or in person at your vet centre.

Our knowledge and understanding of cats – and therefore our ability to look after them in the best way possible – will only improve through our continued research into their anatomy, behaviour and the ways in which their bodies work.

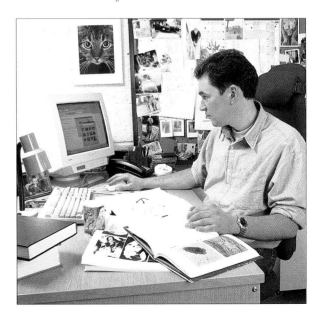

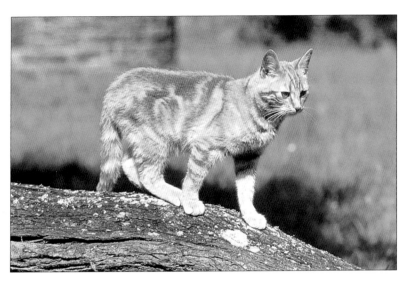

Pet cats have retained many of their wild instincts. They are intelligent and independent: qualities that, combined with their loving natures, make them ideal pets for many owners.

Using this book

When your cat is unwell, your concern for his welfare may be no less than it would be if a human member of your family were either ill or injured. In fact, in my experience, owners are often more worried when their cats are unwell than they would be if they were ill themselves, and there is no doubt in my mind that this worry is often fuelled by a feeling of helplessness.

The aim of this book is to encourage you to take a more pro-active role in your cat's medical care. The better informed you are about common cat ailments – including their major causes and symptoms, and the most up-to-date veterinary procedures available to diagnose and treat them, the better able you will be to make healthcare choices on behalf of your cat. The first section of this book explains the importance of monitoring your cat's health status regularly, in order to identify at an early stage the signs and symptoms of ill-health. When your cat is off-colour, prompt action on your part will prevent him from suffering unnecessarily, and could even save his life.

It may surprise you to discover that – in the UK at least – no-one seems to know for certain what the most common medical conditions suffered by cats actually are. As a result, the conditions that are included in this book have been based on the combined opinions of 180 veterinary surgeons employed by the People's Dispensary for Sick Animals (PDSA).

When your cat is ill, you may find it difficult to absorb at the time (or to remember in detail later on) all the specific information and advice dispensed by your vet or a veterinary nurse. In my experience, even the most level-headed owners can show an understandable lack of mental clarity when their thoughts are clouded by overriding concerns for their cats' welfare. The second section of the book is intended to be considered in conjunction with the specific advice offered by the staff at your vet centre. It will help you to understand not only the condition from which your cat may be suffering, but also the diagnostic procedures and treatments to which he may be subjected, and the kind of nursing care that he is likely to need from you at home.

Choosing the right vet centre is an essential step in providing your cat with the very best in healthcare. As you might expect, vet centres vary considerably, not only in the services that they offer, but also in how they deliver them. It is up to you to find the vet centre in your local area that will best serve you and your cat. Some vet centres treat only cats, while others treat other animals too but are beginning to run special clinics for cats. You will find information on choosing and using vet centres in section three.

The section on special care covers some of the most common practical nursing tasks involved in caring at home for the medical needs of ill or ageing cats, from administering medicines to changing simple dressings. As some of the conditions often suffered by cats are to a large degree preventable, this section also puts into focus the importance of preventive healthcare. With the guidance of the staff at your vet centre, you should devise a preventive-healthcare campaign that is tailor-made to your cat's needs.

If your cat – or someone else's cat – is involved in an accident or other emergency situation, and you are the first person on the scene, being able to carry out basic first aid could save his life. The first-aid section at the end of the book is a quick reference guide to what to do in some of the most common accidents and emergencies affecting cats. You should familiarize yourself with that section now, before you even put this book down: you never know when you may suddenly need to refer to it.

Signs and symptoms

A tail held high, pricked ears and easy, graceful movements are all signs of a healthy cat. Any changes in your cat's behaviour or physical appearance may be symptoms of illness, and recognizing these early by carrying out regular and thorough health-checks may be the key to helping him to a speedy recovery.

Identifying symptoms

Together with your vet, you are an essential part of your cat's healthcare team. This means not only keeping him as healthy as possible by feeding him a balanced diet, encouraging him to take the right sort of exercise, and ensuring that through play and other activities he remains mentally stimulated and happy, but also carrying out a preventive-healthcare campaign of parasite control and vaccination.

It is also important to monitor your cat's behaviour, to record his inputs (food and water consumed) and outputs (urine and faeces produced), and to carry out routine examinations of his anatomy to ensure that you identify any symptoms of disease as soon as they appear. Then, if your cat does become unwell, you will be able to take prompt and appropriate action on his behalf to ensure that he does not suffer unnecessarily.

BEHAVIOUR

A change in your cat's behaviour may be the first sign that he is unwell. If he is grooming himself more than normal, there may be a problem with his skin; if he does not jump on to your lap as usual, it could be that something hurts. Never ignore changes in your cat's behaviour, no matter how trivial they seem.

INPUTS AND OUTPUTS

Changes in your cat's normal drinking, eating and toileting habits may be the result of a number of medical and psychological conditions.

Food

Changes in appetite are a common sign of illness in cats. An increased appetite – particularly in a middle-aged or an older cat – may be significant, especially if he is losing weight at the same time.

Water

The minimum daily water requirement – obtained through eating and drinking – of a healthy adult cat is calculated as 40–70 ml (1½–2½ fl oz) per 1 kg (2¼ lb) of his body weight each day. If your cat is spending more time than normal at his water bowl, keep him indoors and measure his intake over a 48-hour period.

Urine and faeces

Get to know your cat's toileting habits, and the nature of what he usually produces. If he suddenly seems to be relieving himself in unusual places – such as in the open – he may well have a bowel or bladder problem. If you notice these symptoms, keep him indoors for a few days with a litter-tray and see what he produces.

ANATOMY

You should aim to carry out a basic health-check on your cat every week. Once you have established a routine, these checks should only take a few minutes.

The best advice that I can give about health-checks is to be methodical: it does not matter in what order you carry them out, provided that you do not miss anything. At first, you will probably find these checks easiest with your cat on a table. Never put yourself or anyone else in danger: if your cat becomes aggressive when you try to examine him closely, stop and arrange for him to be checked by your vet.

Use your fingers and your nose, as well as your eyes, to gain information about your cat's condition. For instance, the first sign of an ear infection may be a change in the odour wafting from deep inside his ear hole, while the tiny scabs that develop in many skin problems are often easier to feel than to see.

Simple checks

To examine your cat, run your hands firmly over his body, including his legs, stomach and tail. Part the fur and look at the skin: it should be free from flakes and scales. Check for unusual lumps or bumps under the skin. As you move your fingers along his chest, you may be able to feel your cat's heartbeat. If so, count the beats. Most healthy cats at rest have a heart-rate of between 100 and 180 beats per minute. Watch him breathing: the respiratory rate of a cat at rest is usually between 20 and 30 breaths per minute.

Watch your cat's reactions as you palpate him: a quick turn of his head may be the only indication that you have touched on a painful spot. Is he purring, and does he normally purr like this when you stroke him?

WEIGHT-WATCHING

An average adult cat weighs about 4 kg (8¾ lb). A good indication that your cat is at his ideal weight is if you can feel his ribs but not see them. If you cannot feel his ribs, or he has a flap of skin between his hindlegs, he is overweight. By weighing your cat every week you will quickly notice any weight loss or gain, either of which could indicate potentially serious problems.

Remember that a cat who is in severe pain may purr continuously, as well as one who is contented.

Having completed your overall examination, take a closer look at specific parts of your cat's body, using the pictures below as a checklist.

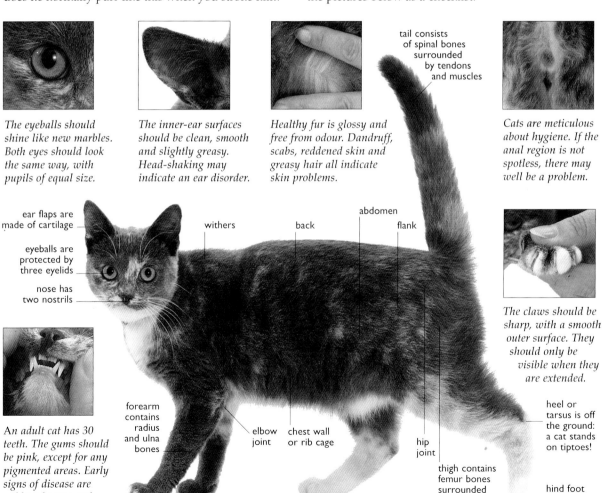

The eyeballs should shine like new marbles. Both eyes should look the same way, with pupils of equal size.

The inner-ear surfaces should be clean, smooth and slightly greasy. Head-shaking may indicate an ear disorder.

Healthy fur is glossy and free from odour. Dandruff, scabs, reddened skin and greasy hair all indicate skin problems.

tail consists of spinal bones surrounded by tendons and muscles

Cats are meticulous about hygiene. If the anal region is not spotless, there may well be a problem.

ear flaps are made of cartilage

eyeballs are protected by three eyelids

nose has two nostrils

withers · back · abdomen · flank

The claws should be sharp, with a smooth outer surface. They should only be visible when they are extended.

An adult cat has 30 teeth. The gums should be pink, except for any pigmented areas. Early signs of disease are reddened gums and brown marks on teeth.

forearm contains radius and ulna bones

forefoot has five clawed toes

elbow joint · chest wall or rib cage

hip joint

thigh contains femur bones surrounded by powerful muscles

heel or tarsus is off the ground: a cat stands on tiptoes!

hind foot has four clawed toes

Reference table of common symptoms

This table is a guide to the conditions covered in the book, and to some of the symptoms most commonly associated with them. The conditions are ordered by parts or systems of the body. There are a number of conditions, including cancer, hyperthyroidism and obesity, that do not fit under the major headings: these are grouped together as 'other important conditions'.

Use this table as a quick index to the conditions in this book and to familiarize yourself with some of the most important symptoms relating to each condition covered. However, avoid the temptation to use the table as a home-diagnosis chart. If you are concerned about anything to do with your cat's health or welfare, always contact your vet centre for advice.

EYE

Conjunctivitis   12–14
- reddened, weepy
  (discharging) eye
- swollen membranes around eye
- partly closed/swollen eyelids
- excessive blinking
- pawing/rubbing at eye
- head-shyness

Corneal disorders   14–15
- dull spot on otherwise
  shiny cornea
- cloudy cornea
- reddened, weepy eye
- excessive blinking
- head-shyness

Epiphora   16
- weepy eye
- brown staining of fur
  at inner corner of eye

Uveitis   17
- reddened eye
- constricted pupil
- cloudiness within eye
- altered eye colour
- blinking/aversion to light

EAR

Otitis externa   18–20
- head-shaking/ear-scratching
- smelly ear
- discharge from ear
- reddened ear hole/ inner ear flap
- head-shyness

MOUTH

Periodontal disease   22–4
- bad breath
- yellow/brown deposits on teeth
- inflamed/receding gums
- difficulty in eating

Gingivitis-stomatitis   24–5
- bad breath
- difficulty in eating
- reddened gums/mouth lining

DIGESTIVE SYSTEM

Vomiting   26–7
(note: this is itself a symptom)
- abdominal heaving
- restlessness
- nausea: drooling and
  excessive swallowing

Parasitic-worm infestation 28–9
- no obvious symptoms
  in most cases
- worms/segments visible
  in faeces or around anus
- vomiting/diarrhoea
- general debility
- pot-bellied appearance

Digestive-system foreign body 30
- repeated or intermittent
  vomiting/regurgitation
- constipation and diarrhoea

Constipation   31
- no faeces produced
- straining to pass faeces
- restlessness

Diarrhoea   32–3
(note: this is itself a symptom)
- soft or watery faeces and/or
  jelly-like mucus
- frequent defecation/'accidents'
- third eyelids across eyes

HEART

Cardiomyopathy   34–5
- unexpected tiredness and
  weakness
- breathing difficulties
- reluctance to eat
- depression
- hindleg lameness or paralysis

AIRWAYS AND CHEST

Chronic bronchial disease 36
- dry cough (often long-term)
- bouts of coughing

Exudative pleurisy   37
- increased breathing rate
- dullness and depression
- weight loss

Feline viral upper-respiratory-
  tract disease ('cat 'flu') 38–9
- sneezing/nasal discharge
- reluctance to eat
- reddened and swollen eyes

Chronic rhinitis   40–1
- 'mucky' nasal discharge
- occasional sneezing

JOINTS, LIGAMENTS AND BONES

Arthritis   42–3
- swollen, painful joint
- lameness
- decreased athleticism
- stiffness, especially after rest
- muscle wastage

Joint dislocation   44
- inability to close jaw properly
- lameness (may be severe)
- resentment of handling
- obviously swollen joint

Bone fracture   45
- painful swelling over affected bone(s)
- obvious wound in some cases
- abnormal appearance to affected body part
- inability to use affected part of skeleton (e.g. broken leg carried)

Lameness   47
(note: this is itself a symptom)
- reluctance to bear weight on affected limb
- excessive grooming of leg

SKIN AND COAT

Alopecia   48–9
- bald areas in coat
- hair-thinning
- itchiness
- skin scaling (dandruff)

Dermatophytosis 'Ringworm'   49
- small, circular bald areas, especially on head, ear flaps and paws; these may contain broken hairs and dandruff

Eosinophilic granuloma complex   50
- ulcerated lips
- swellings/nodules on lips
- nodules on thighs
- red, moist raised plaques on abdomen/inner thighs

Fur mats   51
- tangled hair found anywhere on cat's body, but especially on hindlegs, between toes and in under-tail area

Hypersensitivity reactions   52–3
- intense itchiness
- self-inflicted skin damage
- crusty lumps

Fleas and other skin parasites   54–8
- itchiness (not in all cases)
- self-inflicted skin damage
- some fleas and ticks are visible to naked eye

Miliary dermatitis   58–9
- tiny crusty lumps on skin
- areas of hair loss, containing broken hairs
- restlessness/irritability

Subcutaneous abscess   60–1
- soft swelling (this may rupture, discharging yellow-green pus)
- lameness

Solar dermatitis   62
- reddening of ear tip
- fine scaling of ear tip
- crusty ear tips in more advanced cases

Claw conditions   63
- lameness
- aggression when paw(s) handled
- overlong claws are obvious

KIDNEYS AND BLADDER

Chronic renal failure   64–5
- increased urine production
- increased drinking
- sickness/debility/weight loss (in advanced cases)

Lower-urinary-tract disease   66–7
- frequent urination (and urination in unusual places)
- straining to urinate
- blood-tinged urine

OTHER IMPORTANT CONDITIONS

Cancer   68–9
- very variable symptoms depending on tumour type, size and location
- often general debility

Diabetes mellitus   70–1
- increased urination
- increased thirst
- increased or (more often) decreased appetite
- weight loss
- general debility

Hyperthyroidism   72–3
- increased appetite, but also weight loss
- increased thirst
- hyperactivity (or in some cases depression)
- a change in 'voice'

Ruptured diaphragm   73
- laboured breathing
- lethargy

Liver disorders   74
- Reluctance to eat and weight loss
- depression and lethargy
- abdominal swelling
- jaundice (not in all cases)

Anaemia   75
- lethargy
- reduced appetite and weight loss
- pale gums (can be difficult to tell)
- intolerance of the cold
- rapid breathing on exertion

Obesity   76–7
- physical appearance – ribs cannot be felt easily
- flabby, pendulous abdomen
- lack of normal athleticism and agility

Growing old (ageing)   78–9
many symptoms including:
- swallowing difficulties
- mouth ulcers
- high blood pressure

Common conditions

In this section you will find essential background information relating to some of the most common medical conditions suffered by cats. This is designed to complement the advice that you should obtain from the staff at your vet centre if your cat becomes ill and is suffering from any of these conditions.

Eye

A cat's two eyes are very complex biological cameras. Both they and the tissues that surround them are vulnerable to a large number of conditions, including conjunctivitis, corneal disorders, epiphora and uveitis. If there is any change at all in the appearance of one or both of your cat's eyes, or if you suspect that his sight may be failing – perhaps because he occasionally bumps into objects in unusual places – you must take him to your vet straight away. Any delay could result in him suffering from permanently defective sight.

Conjunctivitis

Conjunctivitis is inflammation of the membrane that lines the inner surfaces of the upper and lower eyelids and covers the exposed part of the eyeball (excepting the transparent cornea). Both sides of the third eyelid are also covered by this membrane.

Conjunctivitis can occur in a cat for numerous reasons, and may be a sudden (acute) condition or a long-term (chronic) problem. It may affect just one of a cat's eyes, or both eyes at the same time.

Causes

Possible causes of conjunctivitis include infection by a bacteria-like organism called *Chlamydia psittaci* (see page 80), or by a bacterial infection (bacteria often become involved in conjunctivitis that was initially due to other causes). Other causes include viral infections – especially feline herpesvirus, but also feline calicivirus – the viruses that are responsible for cat 'flu (see pages 38–9).

Physical irritation can also be a causal factor: for instance, a foreign body (such as a grass seed) may become trapped behind the eyelids. Other causes may include allergies, physical trauma, or eye-anatomy abnormalities such as inadequate tear production or eyelids that are turned inwards.

Other more generalized skin diseases affecting the whole body may also cause conjunctivitis.

Is it serious?

Although it may be uncomfortable, conjunctivitis is not thought to be a very painful condition, as there are few nerves in the conjunctival membranes that are associated with the detection of pain.

Cases of mild, uncomplicated conjunctivitis usually respond well to treatment, but conjunctivitis caused by certain infections may lead to severe problems, especially in kittens or in cats debilitated by

---

COMMON SYMPTOMS

The precise symptoms will depend on the cause of the conjunctivitis, but typical symptoms are as follows:
• Redness of the eye membrane
• Marked swelling of the tissue around the eyeball
• Increased tear production ('crying')
• Excessive blinking

• Half-closed eyelids
• A discharge from the corner of the eye or eyes (this may be watery or thick and 'gooey' in consistency, and grey or green in colour).
• An affected cat may attempt to paw at his eye or rub his face along the ground to relieve irritation.

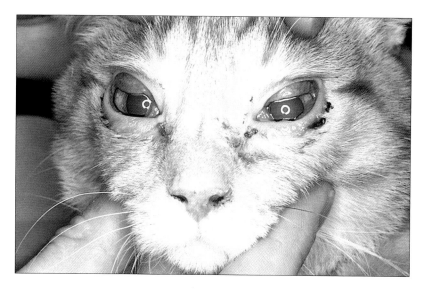

The reddened and swollen membranes around this two-year-old cat's eyes are typical of a case of conjunctivitis.

other illnesses. In some cases, the eyelids may actually stick together and require surgery to be separated. Through pawing at or rubbing his face to relieve irritation, a cat may also quickly cause further damage.

Conjunctivitis caused by feline herpesvirus may recur again and again, despite treatment.

Cats at risk

Cats who roam freely outdoors may be more likely to suffer from eye trauma, or from foreign bodies in their eyes. The area in which a cat lives, the climate and the season of the year – especially in relation to causes such as allergies – may make some cats more prone to suffering from conjunctivitis.

Persian cats with very flat faces have an abnormal eye anatomy that often results in epiphora (see page 16), and possibly, as a result, recurring bouts of conjunctivitis.

Conjunctivitis may be due to infections by certain viruses and *Chlamydia* (see opposite), for which

vaccinations are available, so cats who have not been vaccinated are more likely to be at risk.

Action

If the signs appear very mild – for instance, your cat has watery eyes but does not seem to be in obvious discomfort and is not unwell in any other way – bathe away any tears around his eye or eyes using cotton wool soaked in plain water, or special eye-wipes, and monitor his symptoms. Keep him indoors if possible, as he may pass on an infection to other cats, and any eye discharge will attract debris.

If your cat's symptoms become more severe – for instance, if one or both eyes show signs of redness, or if the tears turn into a mucky discharge – take him to your vet as soon as possible. If his symptoms remain mild, keep monitoring the situation. If your cat is not totally back to normal within three days, contact your vet centre.

Kittens usually suffer from the most severe effects of conjunctivitis, and so should be examined and treated by a vet as soon as possible, even if their symptoms are mild.

Your vet will examine your cat to gain an impression of his general health, before looking at his eyes through an ophthalmoscope (see page 91). He or she may carry out further diagnostic tests, including laboratory analysis of swabs and scrapings taken from your cat's conjunctiva, and tear-production tests (see page 16).

Treatment

If your vet is able to identify the cause of the conjunctivitis, he or she will institute appropriate therapy, such as removing a foreign body.

Even if the precise cause cannot be found at this stage, your vet is likely to prescribe medication that he or she has previously found to be effective: this may include antibiotics, which will need to be continued for at least five days, and/or anti-inflammatory eye ointment or drops (these may be combined in the same preparation). Antibiotics for administration by mouth may be prescribed for conjunctivitis caused by *Chlamydia*, and may be needed for several weeks (see pages 101–2).

No specific treatment is routinely available against any of the viruses that may cause conjunctivitis. As a

ZOONOSIS

People can become infected by the *Chlamydia* organisms (see page 80), but there is very little conclusive evidence that the strain of *Chlamydia* that is responsible for causing conjunctivitis in cats is able to affect us. However, if your cat is diagnosed as suffering from *Chlamydia* infection, you should take sensible hygiene precautions, such as washing your hands using antibacterial soap after handling your cat or cleaning up after him.

result, the aim of treatment in viral infections is to give an affected cat's own body the chance to recover naturally. This is done by helping to control his symptoms, as well as any subsequent bacterial infections that may develop.

Aftercare

At home, you will be responsible for administering the prescribed medication to your cat, so make sure before leaving your vet centre that you know exactly what to do (see also pages 101–3).

You must also keep your cat's eyes clean and prevent him from causing further damage: you may need to fit him with an 'Elizabethan collar' (see opposite, below) for a few days. You should keep him indoors until he has recovered.

Prevention

As part of your cat's day-to-day grooming routine (see page 51), you should regularly wipe away any tears or other debris that accumulates at the corners of his eyes, using special eye-wipes.

All cats should be vaccinated on a routine basis against feline herpesvirus and feline calicivirus (see pages 38–9 and 85).

In addition, any kittens and cats who live in environments in which infection with *Chlamydia* is a known problem should also be vaccinated against infection by this organism. Despite the treatment of those individuals who are showing symptoms, *Chlamydia* infection is very persistent and may remain in affected cat colonies for months or even years.

Corneal disorders

The cornea is the transparent part of the front of the eyeball. It allows your cat to see out and you to see in to the deeper structures of his eye, such as the coloured iris that creates the shape of his pupil.

The cornea is a living part of the eye: its outer layer is completely replaced every seven days.

There are a number of conditions that may affect a cat's cornea. The

most common of these conditions – corneal oedema (the accumulation of water), corneal ulceration and corneal inflammation (also called keratitis) – often occur together.

Causes

Corneal oedema • This may be caused by any disease or injury that affects the delicate structure of the cornea and the process by which water is continually pumped out of it to keep it clear. The presence of abnormal amounts of water within the cornea affects its optical qualities and results in cloudiness. All normal kittens have cloudy eyes when their eyelids open, due to corneal oedema, but this is the only time in a cat's life when it is normal for his corneas to be anything other than crystal-clear.

Corneal ulceration • The causes of this condition may include direct trauma to the cornea (such as that caused by the presence of a foreign body, or by an eyelid that is turned inwards), trauma resulting from dryness due to an inadequate production of tears, and bacterial infection.

Keratitis (inflammation of the cornea) • The main causes of keratitis include infection (for instance, by certain viruses or bacteria), and trauma. It can also occur as a result of other eye conditions, such as uveitis (see page 17). The cause of one particular type of keratitis, known as eosinophilic keratitis, remains unknown.

Is it serious?

In some cases, corneal conditions may resolve spontaneously, or will resolve further to relatively simple treatments. However, any disease affecting a cat's eye should be taken seriously, as it could lead to sight problems if left untreated.

Cats at risk

All cats are at risk of suffering from corneal conditions.

Action

If your cat exhibits any of the symptoms described, take him to your vet as soon as possible.

After giving your cat a complete physical examination, your vet will examine the internal and external

---

COMMON SYMPTOMS

More than one corneal condition may affect a cat's eye or eyes at the same time. He may therefore exhibit a variety of symptoms, depending on the precise cause of the condition and on the degree of the corneal damage. These may include the following:
• Cloudiness of the cornea
• Increased tear production
• Excessive blinking
• Aversion to bright lights
• A red, inflamed eye
• The edges of a corneal ulcer may be visible to the naked eye, although many ulcers are difficult to spot without the use of special equipment and dyes.

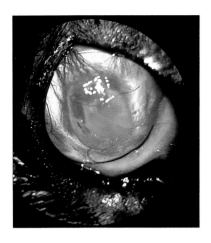

This is the left eye of a cat affected by longstanding corneal ulceration. Blood vessels have grown across the eye in a natural attempt to repair the damage.

features of his eyes with the aid of an ophthalmoscope (see page 91).

In order to highlight a corneal ulcer, your vet may administer a dye called fluoroscein to the cornea. This sticks to most ulcers, but runs off the undamaged corneal surface, and can be made more obvious by illumination with ultra-violet light.

Treatment

The treatment will depend on the severity of corneal damage, and on any identified cause. For instance, if a foreign body is found, your vet will remove it. Other treatment is likely to include the following:

Medication • Unless your cat's cornea is so severely damaged that immediate surgery is required, your vet is likely to begin treatment with antibiotic eye ointment or drops, to keep bacteria at bay while healing takes place naturally. The least severe ulcers will normally heal within one to three days.

In the case of a corneal condition that does not respond to this initial course of medical treatment, more

aggressive measures may need to be taken, such as the following:

Removal of loose corneal tissue • This may be done around the edge of a corneal ulcer, using a dry cotton swab. The procedure will be carried out with your cat under a general anaesthetic (see pages 94–5).

Cauterization • Cauterization, or searing, with specific chemicals may be carried out on the peeling ulcer edges.

Surgery • This may need to be undertaken to fix a flap of healthy conjunctiva across the ulcer; this will protect it and will also place tissue with a good blood supply directly in contact with the area that has been damaged. In most cases, the entire

Fitting an 'Elizabethan collar' (or 'lampshade', as this device is commonly known) to your cat will prevent him from scratching or rubbing at his eye. Your vet or a nurse will select a collar that is the correct size for your cat.

third eyelid will be temporarily sutured across the eye as a patch, but, if a more complex technique is needed, your vet may refer your cat to a specialist.

Aftercare

At home, you must administer the prescribed eye ointment or drops to your cat as directed by your vet (see pages 102–3). You must also keep your cat's eyes clean by gently wiping the inner edges of the eyelids with moist face-wipes. Do not allow your cat outdoors until he has fully recovered. To prevent him from scratching at or rubbing his eye, you may need to fit him with an 'Elizabethan collar' for a few days (see below).

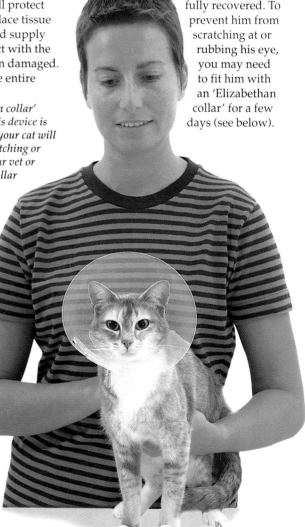

Epiphora

Tears are produced by special glands within the tissues around a cat's eyeball, and normally drain away through the tear duct. This tube is linked internally to the nose, and has two openings in the eyelids at the inner corner of the eye. Epiphora occurs when normal drainage of tears is impeded for some reason, causing the tears to overflow on to the face.

Causes

A cat's tear duct, or the openings into the duct at the inner corner of the eye, may be malformed from birth, making effective drainage of tears impossible.

Alternatively, the duct or its openings may seal up or become blocked later on in a cat's life, due to problems such as infection of the tear duct, a foreign body, excessive mucus collection, or facial injury and subsequent scarring.

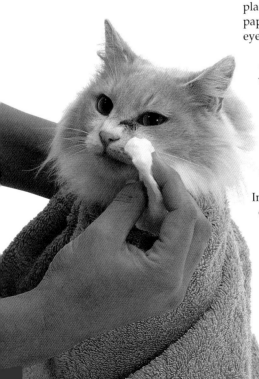

To prevent matting of the fur at the corners of your cat's eyes, and subsequent skin problems, clean away any discharge using damp cotton wool or special eye-wipes.

Is it serious?

Epiphora is not normally serious, unless an infection is involved.

Cats at risk

Epiphora is most commonly seen in breeds with unnaturally flattened faces, especially the so-called ultra- or Peke-faced Persian.

Action

If your cat has a longstanding weepy eye, or obvious tear-staining on his cheek, the effectiveness of his tear-drainage system should be assessed by your vet.

Your vet will examine your cat's eye using an ophthalmoscope (see page 91). He or she will check that the overflow of tears is not due to over-production associated with a condition such as conjunctivitis or a corneal ulcer (see pages 12–15), rather than inadequate drainage.

To confirm this, your vet may place a strip of a special blotting paper behind your cat's lower eyelid: the tears absorbed in a set time can then be compared with figures for normal cats. To check whether the tear-duct openings are blocked, your vet may use a dye called fluoroscein in the eye. If drainage is taking place, the dye will appear at your cat's nostril.

Treatment

In some cases, a blocked tear duct may be cleared by flushing saline or plain water through it.

COMMON SYMPTOMS

Depending on the cause, epiphora may affect one or both eyes, and symptoms that are shown may include the following:
• A constantly weeping eye
• Dark tear-staining or -streaking of the fur close to the inner corner of the eye.
• A red, painful, weeping eye, if the blockage of a tear duct has been caused by infection that has led to conjunctivitis (see pages 14–15).

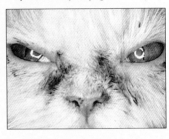

Note the dark-brown staining at the inner corners of this cat's eyes.

This very delicate procedure will be carried out with your cat under a general anaesthetic (see pages 94–5).

If the epiphora is caused by an infection, your vet will prescribe antibiotic eye ointment or drops. In some cases, injections and/or preparations given by mouth may also be required (see pages 101–2).

Surgery to repair a defect in tear drainage is rarely attempted.

Aftercare

If the cause of the epiphora is untreatable, use special eye-wipes or cotton wool soaked in water to clean your cat's eyes regularly.

Prevention

Routine eye-cleaning will remove dirt that could block the tear ducts.

Uveitis

The uvea is a continuous layer of tissue inside a cat's eyeball that envelops the retina and includes the beautifully patterned iris. It is rich in blood vessels.

Uveitis is a condition affecting the eye that is characterized by an inflammation of the uvea. It may occur as a sudden (acute) or a long-term (chronic) condition.

Causes

Uveitis has many possible causes, including physical trauma, cancer (see pages 68–9), immune-system disorders, and infections such as feline immunodeficiency virus infection (see pages 80–2), feline infectious peritonitis (see page 82) and feline leukaemia virus infection (see pages 82–3).

However, in most cases of uveitis the cause remains unidentified despite investigation (see below).

Is it serious?

Uveitis is a very serious condition. It is painful, and in some cases it can cause blindness.

Cats at risk

All cats are at risk of this condition. As certain infectious diseases may cause uveitis (see above), cats who are free-roaming and who regularly have close contact with other cats are likely to be at greater risk.

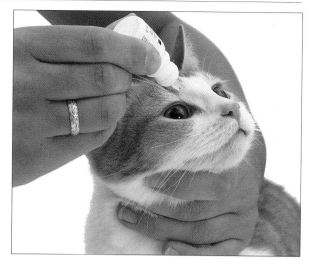

If your cat is suffering from uveitis, you will need to administer eye drops to him at home. Make sure that you know when and how to do this, and how many drops to give on each occasion: full instructions should be on the label (see also page 102).

Action

If your cat exhibits any of the symptoms described, take him to your vet as soon as possible.

Your vet will examine your cat thoroughly before concentrating on his eyes with an ophthalmoscope (see page 91). He or she may use drops of local anaesthetic on the eye (see page 94) to try to confirm whether it is painful. Pressure tests on the eyeball, and blood tests to identify infections, may also need to be carried out.

Treatment

If your vet identifies a specific underlying cause of your cat's condition, he or she will begin any appropriate treatment.

However, in most cases of uveitis the cause cannot be identified or the condition is incurable, so the only possibility is to try to alleviate the symptoms. Eye drops and/or eye ointment to control inflammation and pain are commonly prescribed.

Aftercare

At home, you will need to keep your cat indoors to administer his medication (see pages 102–3). Your vet will wish to see him frequently.

If your cat has been diagnosed as having an incurable disease, such as feline leukaemia virus infection, you will need to make important decisions regarding his future care (see pages 82–3).

Prevention

Uveitis itself cannot be prevented, but you should ensure that your cat is routinely vaccinated against feline leukaemia virus infection.

COMMON SYMPTOMS

Depending on the cause of uveitis, both eyes can be affected but often to different extents. Many symptoms of uveitis are associated with changes inside the eyeball that can only be seen through detailed examination, but a cat may also show the following:
• Reddening of the eye
• A constricted pupil

• Cloudiness within the eye, so that the iris (the coloured part of the eye) does not appear sharply in focus.
• A change in the colour of the iris (due to engorgement with blood).
• Increased tear production, excessive blinking and aversion to bright light.
• Cloudiness of the cornea (see also pages 14–15).

Ear

The most common ear condition to affect cats is inflammation of the skin that lines the external ear canal, or otitis externa. In general, the shape of a cat's ears ensures that his ear canals remain well-ventilated, so that ear wax can dry out rather than accumulating and causing irritation to the lining of the ear. However, if a cat does have irritated ears he will scratch at them, and his claws may inflict severe damage to the ear flaps and nearby skin. If your cat is scratching at or shaking his head, take him to your vet as soon as possible.

Otitis externa

A cat's ear is divided into three parts. The inner ear is housed within his skull, and contains the delicate organs of balance and hearing. The middle ear contains the three ear bones (the malleus, incus and stapes), which transmit sounds to the inner ear from the ear drum. On the far side of the ear drum is the external, or the outer,

ear: this skin-lined tube (called the external ear canal) opens to the outside world at the ear hole.

The most common ear condition to affect cats is an inflammation of the skin that lines the external ear canal. This may occur for many reasons, and is called otitis externa. By scratching at his ear, a cat may quickly cause further problems.

Causes

There are a number of common causes of this condition, including infestation of the ear canal with parasitic ear mites (see page 20), the presence of a foreign body (such as a grass seed) in the ear canal, and infections due to bacteria and yeast living in the external ear canals (these rarely initiate otitis externa, but may complicated cases that are due to other causes).

Other possible causes include more generalized skin conditions such as atopy (see pages 52–3), and cancer (see pages 68–9): as a result of completely or partially blocking the external ear canal, cancerous tumours may predispose the ear canal to infection.

Is it serious?

If it is caught early, otitis externa is not normally a serious condition. However, if it is left untreated it may lead to ulceration of the ear-canal lining, rupture of the ear drum and disease of deeper parts of the ear in the very worst cases.

A cat may also cause severe damage to his ear flap and face by scratching to relieve irritation.

Cats at risk

All cats are at risk of otitis externa. Ear mites (see page 20) seem to be most commonly found in kittens and young adult cats.

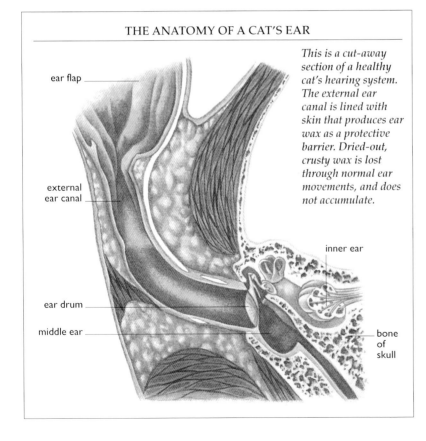

THE ANATOMY OF A CAT'S EAR

ear flap

external ear canal

ear drum

middle ear

inner ear

bone of skull

This is a cut-away section of a healthy cat's hearing system. The external ear canal is lined with skin that produces ear wax as a protective barrier. Dried-out, crusty wax is lost through normal ear movements, and does not accumulate.

Action

If your cat is showing any of the symptoms described, you should arrange an appointment for him to be examined by your vet at the earliest opportunity.

If you are not sure whether your cat's ears are irritating him, gently rub his face under each ear hole in turn, and watch his reaction. If the ear under test is irritating him, he is likely to turn his head on its side with that ear towards the ground and the ear flap flattened, and may rhythmically and rapidly beat his hindleg on that side.

If your cat is head-shaking and scratching frantically he may have a foreign body in his ear canal, and you should contact your vet centre immediately. Do not attempt to clean away any discharge from the ear: this may provide valuable clues as to the cause of the problem.

As a case of otitis externa in your cat may be associated with other, more generalized illnesses (see opposite), your vet should examine the whole of your cat's body as well as his ears. He or she will try to look down the ear canals with the aid of an otoscope (see page 91), but may not see much due to the build-up of wax. Ear mites can also be very difficult to spot, as they run away and hide under pieces of wax as soon as the light from the otoscope reaches the depths of the ear canal.

The cause of the otitis externa may be impossible to identify at this initial examination. If an infection appears to be involved, your vet may take a sample of discharge for laboratory analysis (see page 92). This analysis should identify any organisms that are present, and the medications that should help to bring them under control.

If your vet discovers a tumour or tumours in either of your cat's ear

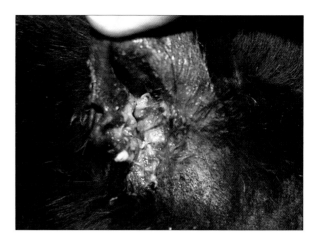

The presence of discharge at either or both of a cat's ear holes is a telltale symptom of otitis externa. This photograph shows an old cat who is suffering from chronic (longstanding) otitis externa.

COMMON SYMPTOMS

Depending on its underlying cause, otitis externa may involve one or both of the ears. Typical signs of this condition include the following:
• A smelly ear or ears
• Discharge from the ear holes: dark brown wax is often indicative of the presence of ear mites (see page 20).
• A reddened ear hole (the inner surface of the ear flap may also show signs of inflammation).
• Vigorous head-shaking

• Excessive ear-scratching, and rubbing of the face along the ground.
• Damage to the ear flap or side of the face, due to self-trauma.
• Resentment of handling or fussing around the ear.

This kitten has an infestation of ear mites (see page 20). The mites have irritated the lining of his external ear canal, causing it to produce copious quantities of brown wax.

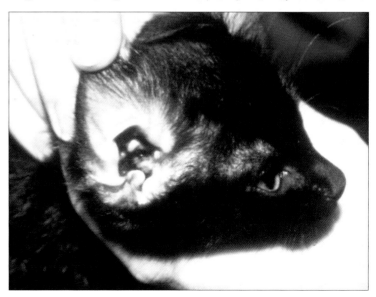

canals, he or she may decide to take some X-ray pictures of his head (see page 91) in order to get an idea of the extent of the tumours.

Treatment

Topical medicine • In a mild case of otitis externa, treatment using appropriate ear ointments or drops is usually effective. Your cat may need more than one kind of topical medicine. For instance, if he has an infestation of ear mites (see right) he will need a drug to kill them, but your vet may also prescribe preparations containing anti-inflammatory drugs to relieve the irritation and to help prevent any further skin damage due to self-trauma. If an infection is a contributing factor to the condition, antibiotic drops or ointments, or anti-yeast drugs, may also be required. The necessary drugs are often mixed together in one preparation.

Ear syringing • In an advanced or more complicated case of otitis externa, the build-up of wax and other debris may be severe. The ear canal may then need washing out for the cause and the extent of damage to the ear-canal lining to be investigated. A clean ear will also allow topical medicines

WARNING

Never put ointment or liquid of any kind into your cat's ear canals, except on the advice of your vet. Without knowing what you are dealing with, you may make your cat's condition worse.

If you poke anything – such as a cotton bud – into his ear canal, you may push back and impact any wax that is on its way out. You could even perforate your cat's ear drum and damage his hearing.

EAR MITES (*OTODECTES CYANOTIS*)

Ear mites are very small, eight-legged, parasitic animals related to scorpions and spiders. They live in the ears of the dog, cat, red fox, racoon, ferret and other meat-eating animals, and may be responsible for over 50 per cent of cases of otitis externa in cats.

Ear mites normally spend their whole lives inside the external ear canal, feeding on skin flakes and debris, but they can survive in the environment for several months. After mating, the adult female ear mites lay eggs that hatch out into larvae. After several moults, in which the tiny creatures completely shed their outer covering to reveal a new one beneath, the males and females mate. The lifecycle from egg to egg takes about three weeks.

A cat is most likely to pick up ear mites through direct contact with an infested animal. The presence of the mites within the ear canals irritates the skin lining the canals, and causes the excessive production of dark brown wax. However, many adult cats appear to develop an 'immunity' to the presence of ear mites. In this case, an affected cat may not exhibit any symptoms associated with the infestation, but he may still pass it on to other cats during close contact.

This is a picture of an ear mite taken under a powerful microscope. These creatures are hard to spot with an otoscope, as they hide from the light.

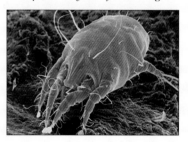

better access to the sites where they are needed. In this case, your vet or a nurse may instill a cleansing solution into your cat's ear while you wait, but, if he resents this or if his ears are very impacted, they may have to be syringed out under a general anaesthetic (see pages 94–5).

Surgery • If your cat's otitis externa is longstanding and there is a permanent thickening of the ear-canal lining, or if it is due to tumours, he may need surgery. A cat may require treatment for a more generalized underlying cause, such as atopy (see pages 52–3), and, in a severe case, medicines may be given by mouth as well as topically.

Aftercare

At home, you must administer any prescribed medication to your cat: this is most likely to involve the frequent use of ear ointment or drops (see page 103). This may need to be continued over several weeks.

In order to prevent your cat from causing further trauma to his ear by scratching or rubbing at it, you may also need to fit him with an 'Elizabethan collar' for the first few days (see page 15).

You will need to clean up any discharge and debris that may accumulate on your cat's affected ear flap, or on the fur around his ear hole, by gently wiping it away using moist face-wipes.

You must keep your cat indoors until he has fully recovered from the infection: your vet will advise you on when this is likely to be. This is to avoid him picking up any dirt and debris in his ears that could complicate his condition, and also to prevent him from passing on the infection to other cats.

Deafness

Deafness is not a condition in itself, but is a symptom of an underlying disorder. Apparent deafness of any duration may be associated with problems in the transmission of sounds to the inner ear via the ear hole, external ear canal, ear drum and bones of the middle ear, or with disorders of the delicate parts of the inner ear that turn sounds into electrical signals. Problems with the nerves that carry these signals away from the ear, or with the parts of the brain in which such signals are interpreted, may also occur.

Deafness may be temporary or permanent, partial or complete, depending on the underlying cause and whether both ears are involved.

Causes

Possible causes of deafness include:
• Blockage of the ear hole or the ear canal: for instance, by a foreign body, by wax or debris associated with otitis externa, or by tumours.
• Rupture of the ear drum.
• A build-up of fluid in the middle ear, due to other ear conditions.
• Abnormalities in the inner ear, associated with ageing.
• Damage to any part of the hearing system, due to trauma.
• An anatomical or a functional abnormality in any part of the

---

COMMON SYMPTOMS

• Lack of an expected response to loud/sudden noises are among the most obvious signs of deafness, but these are often misinterpreted by the cats' owners.
• A cat with only one affected ear may still hear reasonably well, but is likely to lose some of his ability to locate the sources of sounds.

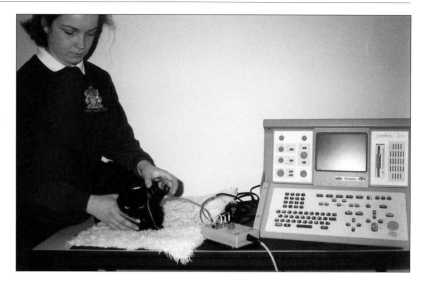

This young cat is being prepared for a hearing test, which will be carried out using equipment designed for people.

hearing system, present at birth, may result in so-called 'congenital' deafness (see below).

Cats at risk

The most common congenital deafness in cats is shown by those with white coats and blue eyes. Charles Darwin apparently said that all white-coated, blue-eyed cats are deaf, but in fact a few do have normal hearing, or only partial deafness. What is more, not all white-coated cats with eyes other than blue have normal hearing.

Action

You can carry out some very simple hearing tests by making sounds of different pitch and intensity from varying locations, and checking your cat's response (make sure that this response is not as a result of sight or feel: hold any noise-making gadget out of sight, and remember that slamming a door may cause a sudden air draught that your cat may feel even if he does not see or hear the door close). If, on the basis

of these tests, you think that your cat may be partially or totally deaf, you should arrange for his hearing to be assessed by your vet.

Your vet will examine your cat's ears to rule out any obvious cause of the apparent hearing difficulty, before carrying out simple hearing tests such as those described. He or she may also arrange an electronic hearing test (if this is available) at a specialist vet centre.

Treatment

Your vet will remove any blockage of the ear hole or ear canal, such as that caused by a foreign body or by otitis externa (see pages 18–20).

If your cat is confirmed as being permanently deaf, try not to worry too much: once you are aware of his disability, you can help him to cope with it. For safety, you may decide to keep him indoors, or restricted to a large outdoor run (see page 40).

Mouth

In my experience, few owners are familiar with the sight of the deeper recesses of their cats' mouths. As a result, many cats with oral conditions are only taken to their vets for attention when symptoms – such as difficulty in eating – become obvious. By this stage, their problems are often well-advanced. Periodontal disease is suffered sooner or later by the vast majority of cats. In order to spot symptoms of oral disease early, you should examine your cat's mouth regularly (see pages 8–9) from the time that he is a young kitten.

Periodontal disease

Periodontal disease literally means disease of the tissues that surround and support the teeth. It is by far the most common oral condition suffered by cats. In the UK, for example, the majority of cats who are over two years old are thought to suffer from at least some degree of periodontal disease.

Causes

This condition is the result of a sequence of events that will have been going on in your cat's mouth since the day on which his teeth first came through.

The outer surface of the teeth is made of enamel, which is the hardest material in the body. In a young cat, this enamel is smooth. Every day the teeth become covered in bacterial plaque, but, through chewing, the plaque is constantly wiped from the smooth enamel. How much remains will depend to some extent on the nature of the cat's diet: for example, some moist foods may tend to stick to the teeth and exacerbate plaque build-up. However, it is still being debated by vets as to whether cats fed on dry food are actually less likely to suffer from periodontal disease.

Plaque is soft, but it rapidly hardens to produce a substance called calculus, or tartar. Unlike enamel, tartar is rough in texture and so plaque is more difficult to remove from it.

COMMON SYMPTOMS

Many of the symptoms of periodontal disease are only obvious on close inspection. By the time that a cat has a problem in chewing, or in closing his mouth, the condition is likely to be very advanced. The following are all common symptoms:
• Bad breath
• Yellow or brown deposits on the teeth at the edges of the gum (these will be rough-looking crusts in an advanced case).
• Reddened gum edges
• Receding gums, revealing exposed tooth roots.

• Drooling saliva (this may be tinged with blood).
• Lack of appetite
• Mouth pain (pawing at the mouth or rubbing the side of the mouth along the ground).
• Difficulty in chewing food.
• Inability to close the mouth.

Amazingly, many cats who have severe periodontal disease manage to continue eating, and owners are often shocked when the extent of the problem is pointed out by their vets during routine health-checks.

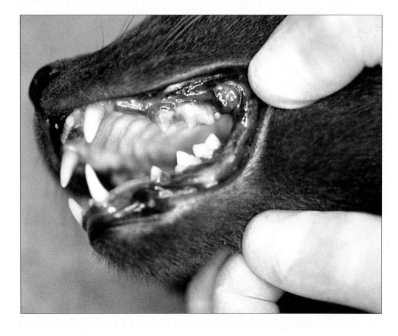

The presence of bacteria in the plaque irritates the gum edges and causes them to become reddened and inflamed: a condition called gingivitis (see pages 24–5). As the gum grows increasingly inflamed, other bacteria start to cause further damage, and the gum may begin to recede around a tooth. Eventually the attachments holding the tooth in place are weakened, and it may then become loose.

The whole process can take several years to complete, but it is reversible in the early stages.

Is it serious?

Advanced periodontal disease is thought to be a painful condition, and is likely to result in tooth loss.

An infected tooth may also act as a reservoir of infection, and any bacteria may find their way from the tooth – via the cat's blood – to his heart, kidneys, liver and lungs, where they may cause disease.

In some cats, periodontal disease may lead on to long-term gingivitis-stomatitis (see pages 24–5).

Cats at risk

All cats are at risk of periodontal disease, although the following may promote its development:
Retained milk teeth • This, or another abnormality of oral anatomy, may encourage food to remain trapped between the teeth; this is thought to promote the build-up of plaque.
Overcrowding of teeth • This condition – to which breeds such as the Peke-faced Persian, with its flat face and small mouth, are prone – encourages food to become trapped between teeth.
Genetics • Some cats seem to fight off periodontal disease better than others. In general, pure-bred cats seem more at risk than cross-bred cats or 'moggies'.

TOOTH-BRUSHING EQUIPMENT

TOOTHPASTES
Toothpastes are made especially for pets, some of which are claimed by their makers to help kill bacteria in plaque. They are palatable and do not froth, and are accepted by most cats.

TOOTHBRUSHES
Special brushes with small heads – made for small puppies – are suitable for use on most cats.

RINSES AND GELS
Special antiseptic rinses, intended to supplement tooth-brushing, are often recommended by vets for use on cats who suffer from recurrent gingivitis. Antiseptic gels are useful for cats who will not tolerate tooth-brushing.

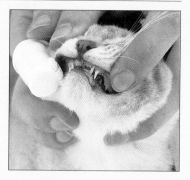

There are many dental-care products available for cats. This rubber glove may be a good training aid, but it is not as easy to use or as effective as a suitable brush. Ask at your vet centre for advice on products for your cat.

Action

Look inside your cat's mouth. If you think that he may be suffering from periodontal disease, take him to your vet centre for a thorough dental check-up.

Your vet will examine your cat's mouth for the obvious signs of periodontal disease. Even if the teeth appear clean and white, your vet will carefully check the gums for inflammation, and may use a disclosing solution to demonstrate any build-up of plaque.

Even if you have a young cat, or an older cat with a set of gleaming white teeth, you should carry out routine dental care by brushing his teeth with a toothbrush and special toothpaste recommended by your vet centre (see above and page 24).

Treatment

The aim of treatment is to remove plaque, tartar and any diseased tissues in order to give the gums a healthier environment.

In a mild case of periodontal disease in which there is little or no build-up of hard tartar on the teeth, the only treatment that is required may be the removal of plaque, through regular tooth-brushing (see above and page 24).

However, no amount of tooth-brushing will remove calculus. If your cat's teeth are encrusted with it, he may need to have it removed by descaling. This will be carried out under a general anaesthetic (see pages 94–5), and involves the use of vibrating instruments that literally shake the deposits from the teeth. With the tartar removed, the enamel is then polished smooth.

In a severe case of periodontal disease, it may be impossible to tell how badly a tooth is affected if it is covered by tartar. If, after the descaling process, your vet finds that one of your cat's teeth is seriously diseased, he or she may need to extract it.

In exceptional cases, a diseased tooth may be saved by advanced dental-surgery techniques (these are normally only available from specialist dentistry centres).

Aftercare

Within just a few days of your cat's teeth being descaled and polished plaque will begin to build up again, so the benefits of any treatment will soon be lost if you do not continue with home dental care. You may not be able to prevent your cat from needing further dental treatment, but you should be able to delay the time when it becomes necessary. Your vet or a veterinary nurse will help you to create a dental-care plan that includes regular check-ups.

Prevention

The key to preventing periodontal disease is the removal of plaque before it hardens into tartar and damages the gum edges. Brushing with special toothpaste is a very effective way of removing plaque, but, if your cat becomes distressed when you try to brush his teeth, do not force him to accept it.

TOOTH-BRUSHING TECHNIQUE

If you have a kitten, you should start handling his mouth in preparation for tooth-brushing as soon as you bring him home: the best time to accustom a cat to this experience is when he is young. If your cat is a wriggler, you may need someone's help to restrain him at first (see pages 98–100).

Initially, simply allow your cat to become used to having his head held and his lips pulled back. Reward his good behaviour immediately with a tiny piece of his favourite food.

Once he accepts this, insert a suitable toothbrush into the pouch formed by his cheek. Hold it there for a few seconds, then remove it. Practise this until your cat is happy with it, rewarding him every time at first and then only intermittently.

When you are both ready, move on to brushing movements, having dipped the brush in water. Hold the brush at an angle of 45 degrees to the

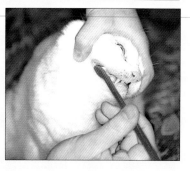

Brushing a cat's teeth is fairly easy if he is well-behaved. If your cat allows you to brush his teeth, aim to do so for about 30 seconds every day.

teeth, and move it gently in an oval pattern. Brush the back teeth at first, then move on to the more sensitive area at the front of the mouth. Only start using toothpaste when you are sure that your cat will tolerate the brushing itself.

Gingivitis-stomatitis

Inflammation of the mouth lining is a common problem. Gingivitis is a localized inflammation of the gums, (most obvious in association with periodontal disease); stomatitis is an inflammation of the whole mouth. These often occur at the same time, and the resulting condition is known as gingivitis-stomatitis. This may take the form of a sudden (acute) condition, but many cats suffer from long-term (chronic) gingivitis-stomatitis that does not respond well to therapy.

Causes

There are many causes of this condition, including the following:
Viral infections • The 'flu viruses, particularly feline calicivirus (see page 38) may be responsible, and

also cause ulcers to appear in an infected cat's mouth. Feline immunodeficiency virus (see pages 80–2) and feline leukaemia virus (see pages 82–3) may also be associated with longstanding cases of gingivitis-stomatitis.
Chemical irritation or traumatic injury • Cats are very selective about what they pick up in their mouths, so will normally only suffer gingivitis-stomatitis for this reason by accident, such as through grooming their coats to remove a substance that is contaminating it (see page 122).
Periodontal disease • The build-up of plaque on teeth will cause gingivitis, and may progress to cause chronic inflammation of large areas of the mouth.

Other major conditions • Serious conditions affecting a cat, such as chronic renal failure (see pages 64–5) or diabetes mellitus (see pages 70–1), may result in the onset of gingivitis-stomatitis. This is because any chronic and debilitating condition may depress a cat's immune system, and will therefore make him more prone to contracting inflammatory mouth disease. Although it is a relatively common problem, chronic and incurable gingivitis-stomatitis often occurs for unknown reasons.

Is it serious?

Chronic gingivitis-stomatitis is a painful condition that is often very difficult to cure or to control.

Cats at risk

All cats are at risk of suffering from this condition.

Action

Smell your cat's breath, and have a look inside his mouth. If he is showing any of the other symptoms described, you should arrange for him to be examined by your vet.

Your vet will examine your cat thoroughly to evaluate his general state of health, and to identify the nature and extent of his symptoms. In an attempt to find the cause of the problem, he or she may decide to carry out further tests, including laboratory analysis of swabs taken from your cat's mouth and blood tests (see page 92).

Treatment

If a treatable cause is identified, your vet will carry out appropriate therapy. For instance, if your cat has severe periodontal disease, he will

COMMON SYMPTOMS

The precise symptoms will depend on the degree to which the cat's gums and mouth are inflamed, and on any specific underlying condition. Typical symptoms may include the following:
• Bad breath
• Difficulty in eating
• Weight loss

• Pawing at the face
• Drooling saliva (this may be tinged with blood)
• Reddened gums and mouth lining
• Symptoms of periodontal disease (see page 22)
• Tacky saliva that stretches across the cat's mouth when it is opened.

need specific dental treatment to resolve it (see pages 22–4).

If a cause cannot be found, your vet will devise a treatment regime that is aimed at controlling your cat's symptoms. This may include antibiotics, although any benefit gained may be shortlived if the underlying cause is not resolved. Anti-inflammatory medicines, such

The lining of this cat's mouth, including his gums, is inflamed and very sore. His symptoms have become chronic because he is infected by FIV (see pages 80–2).

as steroids, (see page 97) may also be used judiciously to help in the control of severe inflammation.

Despite all efforts, chronic gingivitis-stomatitis can be very difficult to control in some cases.

Aftercare

At home, you must administer any prescribed medicines to your cat (see pages 101–2). You may also need to carry out regular oral-hygiene procedures – such as very gentle tooth-brushing or mouth-rinsing – as advised by your vet.

As you would expect, most cats suffering from gingivitis-stomatitis seem to prefer small meals of soft food. Your cat's appetite may also be reduced, so you may have to warm up his food to make it more palatable to him. Ask your vet or a veterinary nurse about a suitable feeding regime: if your cat is only prepared to eat small amounts of food, it is vital that what he does eat fulfils his nutritional needs (see pages 104–5).

Prevention

As gingivitis-stomatitis is often due to periodontal disease, routine dental care at home from an early age should be one of your priorities (see opposite). You must also ensure that your cat is vaccinated against the viruses that cause cat 'flu and feline leukaemia virus infection (see pages 38–9 and 82–5).

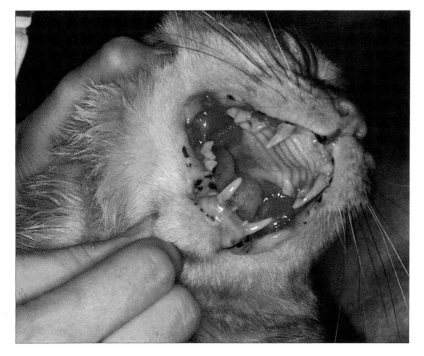

Digestive system

A cat's digestive system acts as a food processor that breaks down food into its component parts before they are absorbed through the bowel wall and used by the body. Any condition that has an adverse effect on the way in which this system works may have serious consequences. Vomiting and diarrhoea are perhaps the most common digestive-system problems suffered by cats. Although vets consider them as symptoms of other conditions, they are included here as specific conditions because that is how most owners perceive them.

Vomiting

Vomiting is a reflex muscular act that results in the forceful ejection of a cat's stomach contents – and sometimes also some of his small-intestinal contents – through the mouth. It should not be confused with regurgitation, which, despite causing a similar end result in some cases, is a much more passive and relaxed act.

Vomiting may occur as a sudden and severe condition, or as a low-grade, chronic complaint.

Causes

Rather than being a condition in its own right, vomiting is associated with many underlying disorders, including the following:
• Sudden changes to the cat's normal diet.
• Ingestion of spoiled food items.

• An intestinal disorder such as a parasitic-worm infestation (see pages 28–9), or an inflammatory large-bowel disease (colitis) that may cause diarrhoea (see pages 32–3) or constipation (see page 31).
• A foreign body in the stomach or intestines (see page 30).
• A food hypersensitivity (see page 53).
• Cancer (see pages 68–9).
• Hormonal disorders such as diabetes mellitus (see pages 70–1) and hyperthyroidism (see page 72).
• A viral infection such as feline panleucopenia (see page 84).
• Poisoning (see page 120).
• A bacterial infection.
• Conditions affecting other major body organs, such as chronic renal failure (see pages 64–5) and liver disease (see page 74).

A cat may also vomit suddenly as a nervous reaction to fear, stress or a change in surroundings, after physical trauma to the head, or due to motion sickness or any other condition that may affect his sense of balance, such as some forms of ear disease.

Is it serious?

Most cases of vomiting are due to inflammation of the stomach lining (gastritis). As this usually responds well to starvation and dietary management, the underlying cause is rarely investigated. However, vomiting can be life-threatening.

The seriousness of each case will depend on its cause, the time since its onset and the frequency of vomiting. Anything other than very occasional, sporadic vomiting of known cause should be considered potentially serious. Severe and frequent vomiting is an emergency.

Cats at risk

All cats are at risk of vomiting.

Action

If your cat vomits unexpectedly, keep him indoors, observe him carefully and do not offer him food or water for at least four hours.

If he does not vomit again, treat him as normal, but keep him in with a litter-tray for 24 hours to observe him and to check whether he has diarrhoea (see pages 32–3).

COMMON SYMPTOMS

• Vomiting within minutes or up to a few hours after eating may be the only or the main symptom of some conditions, such as acute gastritis (inflammation of the stomach wall) after eating spoiled food.
• Persistent vomiting of large volumes of liquid in the face of starvation is typical of a bowel obstruction caused by a foreign body (see page 30).
• Depending on the cause, other symptoms (such as diarrhoea) may be exhibited by an affected cat.

The act of vomiting involves three phases: nausea (the cat may look concerned, lick his lips and swallow repeatedly); retching, as the stomach begins to contract (forceful breathing movements are characteristic of this phase); and vomiting, which involves the co-ordinated movement of the diaphragm and the abdominal-wall muscles. This results in a heaving action that forces the contents of the stomach up the oesophagus and then through the cat's mouth.

If he does vomit again within four hours, withhold food for a further 24 hours, but offer him a few laps of water every 30 minutes. If your cat continues to vomit, if the vomit is very dark-coloured or contains blood, or if he shows other signs of illness, such as lethargy, contact your vet centre straight away.

If your cat does not vomit again within the 24-hour period, offer him unrestricted access to water, but make sure that he does not drink excessively. Feed him a small and highly digestible, low-fat, low-fibre meal of rice with a little hard-boiled egg or chicken, or a prepared diet formulated for cats with digestive disturbances (see page 105).

Continue to offer similar small meals every four hours during the day. If your cat remains well and does not vomit again, gradually mix in his normal food over the next two days.

If you need to take your cat to your vet, he or she will examine him thoroughly, and will ask you specific questions about the timing of the vomiting episodes and the nature of the vomit.

Your vet's aim will be to identify and treat any underlying cause of the vomiting, to replace any lost fluids and to control the vomiting. Diagnostic tests may include blood, urine and faeces analysis, X-ray and ultrasound investigations, and examinations using an endoscope (see page 91).

Treatment

This will depend on the severity of the vomiting, and on any identified cause. Nine out of 10 cases may respond to dietary management alone, but some cases benefit from the use of appropriate medicines.

An intestinal obstruction that is due to a foreign body (see page 30) may need to be resolved by surgery.

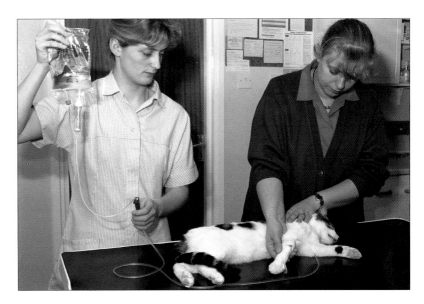

Cases of sudden and severe vomiting need intensive therapy to control the symptoms and to treat the effects of repeated vomiting on body chemistry. If a specific cause is not identified, treatment is likely to consist of nothing given by mouth for 24 to 48 hours, and immediate treatment with fluid via an intravenous drip (see page 93) until the cat can take in sufficient water by mouth. Drugs may be used to control vomiting, thereby resting the digestive system and preventing further loss of fluids.

Appropriate on-going dietary management should be instigated as soon as the cat is able to keep down food.

Aftercare

Your cat may need to remain at your vet centre as an in-patient for tests or treatment, particularly if he is very unwell. When he returns home, you should keep him in until he has fully recovered, continue the administration of any prescribed medicines (see pages 101–2), and carry out the specific dietary advice that you are given.

Repeated vomiting will quickly result in dehydration, so giving fluids via a 'drip' (see page 93) may save a cat's life.

Prevention

It may be impossible to prevent many of the specific causes of vomiting, but the following are sensible precautions:
• Keep your cat's vaccinations up to date (see page 85).
• Base his diet on high-quality prepared cat foods (ask at your vet centre for advice).
• If your cat has a big appetite, offer him his daily food allowance split into several meals. Studies have shown that many cats are 'snack' feeders, and that some prefer to eat 10 meals or more per day.
• Do not make any sudden changes to your cat's diet.
• Do not feed him your left-overs.
• Routinely treat him for intestinal worms (see pages 28–9).
• Groom him regularly if he has a long coat, in order to prevent him from ingesting excessive amounts of hair through self-grooming.
• Do not feed your cat just before travelling with him in the car.

Parasitic intestinal-worm infestation

Parasites are organisms that live in or on other animals and derive their nourishment from them. A number of parasitic worms may live and reproduce within a cat's intestines, but the most common of these are tapeworms and roundworms.

TAPEWORMS

There are two types of tapeworm that may affect cats in the UK.

Dipylidium caninum • These worms are flat, white and consist of many segments. They can grow up to 50 cm (20 in) long, but most reach a length of about 20 cm (8 in). They may be present in large numbers: up to 100 have been recorded. Segments of an adult tapeworm, containing worm eggs, break off in a cat's intestines and leave his body via his anus. The segments then release their eggs. An immature flea (or, less commonly, a louse) in the environment may eat these eggs, which will continue to develop inside the flea's body. As an adult, the flea will search for an animal to jump aboard to suck blood: this may be the same or another cat (or even a dog or a person). As it feeds the flea will create irritation, causing the cat to nibble and groom his skin. In doing so, he may swallow the flea, which will be digested and release immature tapeworms into the cat's intestines. And so the cycle continues.

Taenia taeniaformis • Normally only three or four of these worms are present in a cat's intestines at one time, but each may be up to 30 cm (12 in) long. With this tapeworm, rodents – such as rats, mice and voles – take the place of fleas or lice in the lifecycle, so this tapeworm is normally only a problem in habitual hunters.

Tapeworm infestations rarely cause severe problems in cats, unless the worms are present in very large numbers. However, as people can be infested by *Dipylidium caninum* (see above, right), a tapeworm

COMMON SYMPTOMS

Infestations with tapeworms most commonly affect older kittens and adult cats. They may go unnoticed, but common symptoms include the following:
• White segments wriggling about on the fur around the cat's anus, on his bedding or on the ground.
• An affected cat may spend a lot of time grooming his bottom.
• Digestive disturbances, such as diarrhoea (see pages 32–3).
• General lethargy and debility.

ZOONOSIS

Although it is extremely unlikely, it is possible for people to become infested with *Dipylidium caninum* tapeworms. While playing with your cat, for example, a member of your family could swallow a flea, concealed in his fur, that contains eggs. Once digested, the worm would be able to develop inside that person's intestines.

infestation must be taken seriously. Assume that your cat is infested and, using a wormer recommended by your vet, dose your cat as soon as he comes to live with you, and at appropriate intervals (see page 112). Wormers are normally given by mouth (see pages 101–2). Your prevention campaign should also include flea control (see page 56).

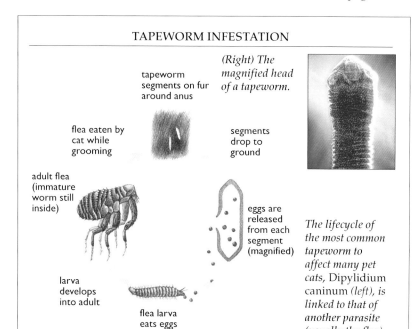

TAPEWORM INFESTATION

tapeworm segments on fur around anus

(Right) The magnified head of a tapeworm.

flea eaten by cat while grooming

segments drop to ground

adult flea (immature worm still inside)

eggs are released from each segment (magnified)

larva develops into adult

flea larva eats eggs

The lifecycle of the most common tapeworm to affect many pet cats, Dipylidium caninum *(left), is linked to that of another parasite (usually the flea).*

ROUNDWORMS

The most important intestinal roundworm of cats in the UK is *Toxocara cati*. Adult roundworms of this type may grow up to 15 cm (6 in) long, and live in an infested cat's small intestine.

A cat may become infested with *Toxocara cati* roundworms in the following ways:

As a kitten • Immature worms that have developed from eggs eaten by a kitten's mother appear in her milk during lactation. These are swallowed, develop into adults and lay eggs that pass out in the kitten's faeces.

In the environment • Eggs passed out in faeces take several weeks to develop to a stage at which they can infest another cat. If they are swallowed by a kitten, the eggs develop in the intestines into adult worms; in adult cats they hatch and immature worms go to other tissues, where they become dormant. (It is unusual for adult worms to be present in an adult cat's intestines.)

By eating other animals • If eggs are eaten by an earthworm, beetle, rodent, rabbit or bird, immature roundworms hatch out, find their way into its body tissues and become dormant.

COMMON SYMPTOMS

There are often no signs at all, but a heavy infestation in a kitten of less than eight weeks old may cause the following symptoms:
• Diarrhoea (see pages 32–3)
• A poor coat
• General debility
• A pot-bellied appearance
• Adult worms are occasionally vomited, or may be passed as a tangled knot in a kitten's faeces (in a severe infestation).

Through hunting any of these infested animals, a kitten or cat may himself become infested. The immature worms are then released during digestion and develop into egg-laying adults. Roundworm infestations can cause severe illness, especially in young kittens. The worms can also affect people (see right).

If you have a kitten who was not wormed by his breeder in his first weeks (see page 112), he will almost certainly have roundworms. You should assume that he is infested, and start a prevention campaign.

All kittens and cats should be wormed regularly (see page 112). Wormers are available in various forms, including liquids, tablets and granules, and are given by mouth or in food (see pages 101–2).

Remove and dispose of faeces from litter-trays or your garden promptly, so that roundworm eggs do not have time to develop to the point at which they can infest a cat.

ZOONOSIS

Roundworms can affect people if they pick up eggs on their hands from the environment and then accidentally swallow them (it is unlikely that a person would pick up eggs capable of infesting them by touching a cat, as the eggs take several weeks to reach that stage).

Inside a human's intestines the eggs will hatch. Immature worms may cause damage and disease as they move around their bodies, but medical problems caused by *Toxocara cati* are thought to be rare. The following are important ways of reducing the chance of human infestation still further:
• Children should be taught good basic-hygiene habits, and should wash their hands before eating.
• Food should be covered to prevent contamination by flies.
• Cats should be encouraged to defecate in litter-trays, and faeces should be cleared up immediately.

ROUNDWORM INFESTATION

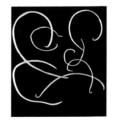

Toxocara cati *roundworms (above) have pointed, cream-coloured bodies.*

The major sources of roundworm infestation in young kittens and cats (right).

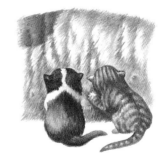

kittens become infested through drinking milk

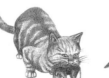

kitten or cat becomes infested by eating prey

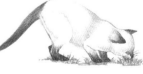

kitten or cat becomes infested by picking up eggs in environment

Digestive-system foreign body

A foreign body is any object that is in an abnormal place. In terms of a cat's digestive system, a foreign body is any solid object that is not considered a food item. Typical examples include hair balls, string or sewing thread, fishing hooks and bone fragments.

Causes

Unlike dogs, cats are generally very selective about what they pick up in their mouths, but they may inadvertently swallow a foreign body when playing or hunting.

For example, almost all kittens and most adult cats enjoy playing with dangling objects such as wool or cotton threads. If your cat sees a piece of thread hanging out of your sewing box, he is likely to have a go at pulling it. However, once in his mouth, the thread will be difficult for him to spit out because of the backward-pointing barbs on his tongue. As a result, he may swallow the thread (and eventually any needle that may be attached to it).

Is it serious?

A foreign body may pass right through a cat's digestive system without causing any problems, but another – such as a fishing hook – could become impaled in his oesophagus, stomach or intestines.

A large, irregularly shaped or rough-textured foreign body – such as a piece of bone or a matted hair ball – could partially or completely block the digestive system with life-threatening consequences.

Cats at risk

All cats are at risk, although some cats seem particularly attracted to eating unusual objects. For instance, fabric-eating is a well-known behaviour abnormality of the Siamese and Burmese breeds, and of other oriental types. Precisely what stimulates these cats to do this is not known.

Action

If you think or know that your cat has swallowed a foreign body, or if he shows any of the symptoms described, keep him indoors and contact your vet centre as soon as possible. Do not allow your cat to take anything by mouth until you have spoken to your vet.

Your vet will examine your cat thoroughly. Depending on how unwell he is, on the history of his illness and on the findings of this examination, your vet may also carry out X-ray and ultrasound investigations (see pages 91–2).

COMMON SYMPTOMS

A foreign body may cause a cat problems if it becomes lodged in his oesophagus, in his stomach or in his intestines. The symptoms will depend on the location of the foreign body, the irritation that it causes and the degree to which it blocks the digestive system, but typical symptoms may include any of the following:
• Excessive drooling (especially when a foreign body is obstructing the oesophagus).
• Regurgitation and/or vomiting (see pages 26–7): this may go on for several weeks in the case of a partial obstruction.
• Lack of appetite
• Debility and dehydration
• Abdominal swelling, due to gas build-up in the intestines.
• Constipation or diarrhoea
• Weight loss (in a chronic case)

Treatment

Your vet may observe your cat for a period, or may decide to operate straight away. If your cat has been vomiting, he may require fluids given through an intravenous drip (see page 93), and he will almost certainly be given antibiotics.

If the foreign body is stuck in your cat's oesophagus, surgery to remove it may be carried out using an endoscope (see page 91); if this is unsuccessful, he may need open-chest surgery.

A foreign body lodged in his stomach or intestines will probably be removed through a small hole in the wall of his gut. If a piece of his bowel has been damaged, your vet may need to remove it.

Aftercare

After surgery, your cat will need to stay in at your vet centre for intensive nursing. Your vet will only discharge him when he is well on the way to recovery.

At home, you should keep your cat indoors and nurse him until he has recovered (see pages 98–111). You will need to administer any prescribed drugs, and to follow the specific feeding advice that you are given. You must also monitor your cat's food intake, disposition and bowel movements, and take him for post-operative check-ups.

Prevention

Never leave your cat unsupervised with objects (including toys) that he may be able to swallow, and avoid offering him any food that may contain small cooked bones. Brush him regularly to prevent him from ingesting excessive amounts of hair through self-grooming.

Constipation

A cat is constipated if he defecates less frequently than usual, or not at all. The number of times a day that a normal cat defecates will depend on his diet and feeding regime, as well as on the personal peculiarities of his digestive system.

Causes

Constipation has various causes, including the excessive ingestion of hair, a blockage of the intestines by a tumour or a foreign body (see opposite), and obstruction of the passage of faeces due to a pelvic fracture. Nerve damage due to 'tail-pulling' injuries, a debilitating disease that results in inactivity, and pain during defecation may also cause constipation.

In some middle-aged and older cats, the muscular wall of the large bowel fails to contract normally and becomes distended with faeces. The cause of this is unknown.

Is it serious?

This depends on the precise cause of the constipation (see above).

Cats at risk

Some cats may be constipated on just one occasion; others may suffer frequently as a result of permanent disabilities such as pelvic fractures or nerve damage, and may require long-term preventive management.

Action

If your cat always defecates in a litter-tray, you should soon notice if he is constipated. Even if he goes to the toilet outside, it is a good idea to provide him with a litter-tray indoors. If he becomes constipated, or suffers from any other bowel disorder, he may begin to use the tray unexpectedly.

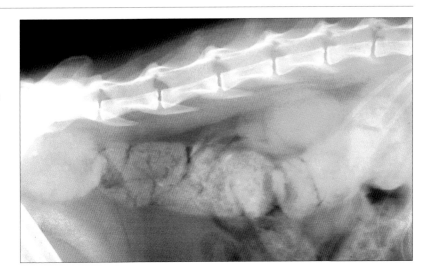

If you are in any doubt as to your cat's toileting habits, keep him indoors with a litter-tray until he produces something. However, a word of warning: some cats become constipated due to confinement!

If your cat suddenly suffers from constipation, you should take him to be examined by your vet. In order to identify the cause and the seriousness of the constipation, your vet will give him a thorough physical check-up, including a rectal examination and abdominal palpation. He or she may also carry out blood tests, abdominal X-rays and an ultrasound examination (see pages 91–2).

COMMON SYMPTOMS

- The production of less faeces than normal, or none at all.
- The production of very dry and hard faeces.
- Straining during attempts to defecate.
- Restlessness
- General debility

The build-up of faeces in the bowel of this constipated cat appears as a string of grey objects on this X-ray picture.

Treatment

Therapy for constipation involves relieving the symptoms, treating the cause (where possible) and instituting measures to prevent recurrence (see below).

Symptomatic therapy may include the administration of laxatives, or of enemas to remove impacted faeces. Fluid therapy may also be given, via an intravenous drip (see page 93).

Prevention

The most appropriate preventive measures will depend on the cause of the constipation. These may include more frequent grooming of your cat to remove loose hairs that he could ingest, encouraging more activity, and adding bulk-forming laxatives (such as bran) or faecal softeners to his diet. A better option may be to offer him a prepared diet specially formulated for cats with constipation (see page 105).

Diarrhoea

Diarrhoea in a cat is a symptom of other underlying disorders – most commonly directly involving the digestive system – rather than being a condition in its own right. It may be a symptom of any disease that reduces the ability of a cat's bowel wall to absorb fluid, stimulates it to pour more fluid than normal into his digestive system, or adversely affects his bowel movements.

Diarrhoea is most obvious as the production by a cat of unusually watery faeces, although a cat who defecates more frequently or produces larger volumes of faeces than normal may also be described as suffering from diarrhoea.

Causes

Causes of diarrhoea include dietary upsets (for example, due to sudden changes to the usual diet), bacterial infections, and viral infections such as feline panleucopenia and feline leukaemia virus infection (see pages 82–4).

Intestinal-worm infestations (see pages 28–9), food allergies, and conditions such as renal failure (see pages 64–5), hyperthyroidism (see page 72) and liver disease (see page 74), as well as psychological upsets, may also be responsible.

Chronic, or long-term, diarrhoea is a fairly common problem in cats. Although most cases will respond sooner or later to symptomatic treatment, the cause of diarrhoea often remains unidentified.

Is it serious?

Most cases of sudden diarrhoea are mild and will respond well to symptomatic treatment. However, some acute cases of diarrhoea – such as those that are associated with feline panleucopenia – may

be life-threatening. It can also be very difficult to manage chronic diarrhoea, so the sooner this is investigated by a vet, the better.

Diarrhoea in a kitten may lead on to a life-threatening condition called intussusception, in which one piece of bowel telescopes inside another. An affected kitten will begin to vomit, and will die if the intussusception is not corrected. In most cases, this requires surgery.

No matter what the history, all cases of diarrhoea should be taken seriously until proved otherwise.

Cats at risk

All cats are at risk of diarrhoea, but kittens and also old cats seem particularly vulnerable to diarrhoea due to certain causes.

Young kittens • Diarrhoea is very common in kittens separated from their mother and litter mates, and may well be due to stress. A kitten may also become infested with roundworms from his mother's milk (see page 29). Kittens seem more prone than adult cats to diarrhoea due to dietary upsets and infections.

Old cats • These cats are most likely to suffer from diarrhoea resulting from chronic renal failure (see pages 64–5) and bowel cancer (see pages 68–9). Symptoms are often vague, and may include a variable appetite, dullness, progressive weight loss and only intermittent diarrhoea.

Action

If your cat suffers from a bout of severe diarrhoea and exhibits any other symptoms such as lethargy or vomiting (see pages 26–7), or he appears to be far from his normal self, keep him indoors and contact your vet centre immediately.

If your cat suffers from a bout of diarrhoea but appears to be in all other respects his normal self, keep him indoors to monitor him and see what he produces, and only give him water for 24 hours. If after this time he still has diarrhoea or begins to show other symptoms, contact your vet centre.

If the symptoms have eased after 24 hours, continue to keep your cat indoors and offer him a small, highly digestible meal of boiled

---

COMMON SYMPTOMS

The symptoms will depend on the cause and severity of the diarrhoea, but may include the following:
• Bulky faeces that are also softer in consistency than normal.
• Large volumes of very watery faeces (these may be very dark in colour, foul-smelling and look as though they contain blood).
• Colour changes to the faeces (normal cat faeces are often black, but may become yellow or green in certain types of diarrhoea).

• Greasy-looking faeces
• Small amounts of faeces, often mixed with jelly-like mucus, produced very frequently. An affected cat may strain to go to the toilet, and may also have toileting 'accidents' indoors: this is typical of inflammation of the large bowel (colitis).
• Pain on defecation
• Abdominal discomfort
• Vomiting (see pages 26–7)
• Weight loss
• Third eyelids partially across eyes.

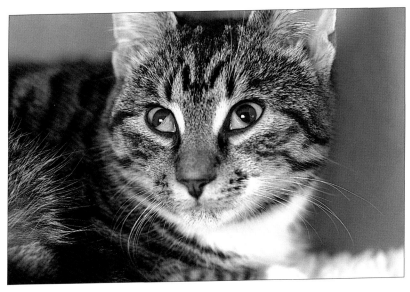

If your cat's third eyelids appear to be permanently partway across his eyes, he may be suffering from diarrhoea.

rice with a little hard-boiled egg or chicken. Better still, offer him a prepared diet formulated for cats with digestive disturbances (see page 105). Continue to offer him similar small meals every four hours during the day, and monitor what he produces.

If your cat has diarrhoea again as soon as you feed him, contact your vet centre. If he remains well and his faeces firm up, gradually mix in his normal food over the next two days until he is back to his normal regime. Only let him outdoors again when he has fully recovered.

If you need to take your cat to your vet, he or she will examine him carefully to try to identify the cause of the diarrhoea. Further investigations may then be needed, including blood tests, analysis of faeces, examinations using an endoscope, X-ray and ultrasound investigations, and microscopic examinations of biopsies of the bowel wall (see pages 91–2).

Treatment

The aim of treatment will be to give your cat's digestive system a rest, to replace lost body fluids and to deal with any identified cause: this may be as straightforward as worming your cat (see pages 28–9), or as complex as instituting therapy for a major condition such as renal failure (see pages 64–5).

Sudden, severe diarrhoea needs intensive therapy to control the obvious symptoms and to treat the effects of fluid loss on body chemistry. Many cases of diarrhoea will resolve as a result of fluid administration and bowel rest; others may require specific medicines. An intestinal foreign body may need to be removed.

If a specific cause cannot be identified, your cat's treatment may include any or all of the following:
• No food given by mouth for 24 to 48 hours.
• Special fluids administered by mouth or directly into the blood via an intravenous drip (see page 93).
• Drugs to help to control his bowel movements.
• Anti-inflammatory medicines.

• Antibiotics in exceptional circumstances (such as when blood in the faeces suggests that the bowel wall is severely damaged).
• After 24 to 48 hours' starvation, the institution of an appropriate dietary regime.

Aftercare

At home, you will need to keep your cat indoors and nurse him (see pages 98–111). You must administer his prescribed medicines, and also implement the dietary advice that you are given by your vet.

Be patient: if your cat is suffering from chronic diarrhoea, it may take several weeks for him to recover.

Prevention

Some of the causes of diarrhoea may not be preventable, but the following measures are all sensible precautions to take:
• Keep your cat's vaccinations up to date (see page 85).
• Feed him on the highest-quality prepared foods that you can afford (see also page 105).
• Do not make sudden changes to his diet: gradually mix in new food with the old for at least two days.
• Avoid giving him your left-overs.
• Offer him cows' milk with care, as many cats – with the exception of very young kittens – cannot digest lactose, one of the sugars in milk.
• If your cat has a big appetite, split his daily food into several meals.
• Treat him routinely for parasitic intestinal worms (see pages 28–9).

ZOONOSIS

Certain bacteria that can cause diarrhoea in cats may also affect people. If your cat has diarrhoea, you and your family should be extra-vigilant about hygiene after handling your cat.

Heart

A cat only remains alive thanks to the unrelenting efforts of just one muscle: his heart. Unfortunately, cats' hearts are vulnerable to a serious condition called cardiomyopathy. As cats can be fairly lethargic animals for much of the time, the earliest symptoms of heart disease – notably tiredness – are often missed, even by the most diligent owners. Untreated cardiomyopathy is a life-threatening condition. To try to identify it early, all cats should undergo a basic heart evaluation as part of routine annual veterinary health-checks.

Cardiomyopathy

This is the most significant cause of heart failure in cats. There are a number of different types of the condition, the most common of which is known as hypertrophic cardiomyopathy. This is associated with a marked thickening of the heart-muscle mass that encloses one of the heart's two larger chambers, the left ventricle. This muscle mass is responsible for pumping blood through the aorta, which is the body's largest artery.

Another condition called dilated cardiomyopathy is associated with weakness of the heart muscle, and is less common.

Causes

Hypertrophic cardiomyopathy may be the result of various problems, including high blood pressure due to renal failure (see pages 64–5) and hyperthyroidism (see page 72). However, in most cases the cause of the condition is unknown.

Dilated cardiomyopathy occurs in cats who do not eat enough of a specific amino acid (a building block of protein), called taurine. This condition is extremely unusual in cats who are fed on high-quality prepared cat foods.

Is it serious?

Cardiomyopathy may be life-threatening but, if a specific cause is identified and resolved, many or all of the changes in the heart can be reversed. Even if the cause is unknown, treatment can alleviate symptoms for long periods.

One serious complication that is associated with cardiomyopathy is that of blood clots settling in the arteries to the hindlegs: this can be difficult to control and to cure.

Some cats with cardiomyopathy die suddenly and unexpectedly.

Cats at risk

Cardiomyopathy occurs mainly in cross-bred cats – especially in those with long hair – for unknown reasons. As many as four times more male than female cats seem to suffer from this condition, and it may affect individuals as young as five months old.

Action

If your cat exhibits any of the symptoms described, you should arrange for him to be examined by your vet as soon as possible.

Your vet will consider the history of the symptoms before carrying out a thorough clinical examination. This process will include the use of a stethoscope to listen to your cat's heart (see page 91).

If your vet considers that your cat may have a heart condition, he or she is likely to carry out X-ray and ultrasound investigations, ECG recordings and blood tests (see pages 91–2). An assessment of your cat's current dietary regime may also be appropriate.

COMMON SYMPTOMS

A normal, healthy cat may sleep for up to 16 hours each day and, because few owners know exactly how much exercise their cats take from day to day, the sometimes vague symptoms associated with cardiomyopathy are easy to miss. Indeed, symptoms can be so vague that cardiomyopathy is often only discovered during routine examinations or investigations into other disorders.

An affected cat may show no obvious symptoms for a time, and may then suddenly deteriorate. The common symptoms of this condition include the following:

• Breathing difficulties (but rarely coughing), due to the accumulation of fluid in the lungs or chest.
• Lack of appetite
• Lethargy and weakness
• Fainting
• Weight loss
• Abdominal swelling
• Vomiting in occasional cases (see pages 26–7).
• Inability to use the hindlegs: an affected cat may also experience pain in the legs, caused by blood clots that form in the diseased heart and then settle in the arteries that supply the hindlegs with blood.

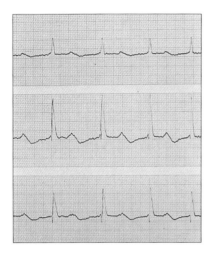

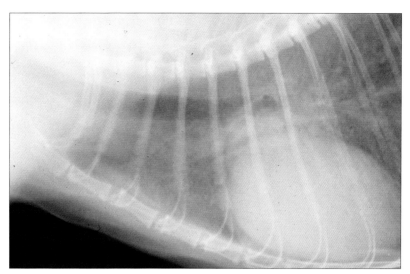

This ECG trace and X-ray (above and right) are from a cat with hypertrophic cardiomyopathy. On the ECG (see also page 92), the tall 'spikes' are typical of the condition, while the X-ray reveals that the heart is greatly enlarged.

Treatment

If your cat's heart is beginning to fail and fluid is building up in his lungs or chest, your vet will treat him with medicines aimed at reducing the workload on the heart and encouraging fluid to drain away from the sites in which it has accumulated. Your cat will need emergency treatment if he has symptoms associated with blockage to the main arteries of his hindlegs.

If further investigations identify an underlying cause, your vet will institute any appropriate treatment. For instance, if your cat is suffering from hyperthyroidism (see page 72) your vet may elect to operate, or to use drugs that are toxic to your cat's thyroid glands. If your cat may be taurine-deficient, he will need taurine supplementation and his diet must be adjusted as necessary.

If the cause of the condition is unknown, your vet will devise a treatment plan using medicines to help the diseased heart.

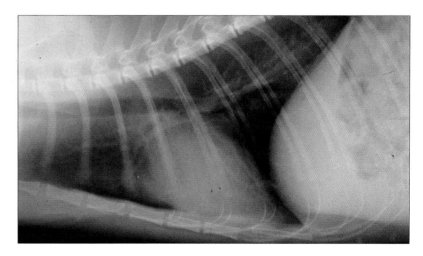

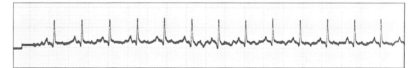

Aftercare

At home, you must administer any medicines prescribed by your vet (see pages 101–2), and follow his or her recommendations as to your cat's general management. For example, if your cat's heart is in failure, you must keep him indoors and well-rested.

Compare the second X-ray picture and the ECG trace (above), which are taken from a normal, healthy cat, with those of the cat suffering from hypertrophic cardiomyopathy. The lemon-shaped heart is considerably smaller in this picture. Most of the remainder of the chest consists of the cat's lungs, which are filled with air and appear as dark areas on the X-ray.

Airways and chest

A cat's airways consist of his nasal cavities, his windpipe and the network of smaller pipes that connect it to many thousands of microscopic chambers within the lungs, where the exchange of oxygen and carbon dioxide to and from the blood takes place.

Cat 'flu, or feline viral upper-respiratory-tract disease, is a serious condition to which all cats are vulnerable and which can lead to chronic rhinitis. Other conditions that affect the airways and chest are exudative pleurisy (pyothorax) and bronchial disease.

Bronchial disease

Cats may suffer from a number of diseases that affect their lower airways, or bronchi, all of which result in obstruction of the normal flow of air in and out of the lungs. These include asthma and also bronchitis, which is characterized by inflammation of the bronchi.

Causes

The underlying cause often remains unknown, but possible factors may include allergies, bacterial infection and exposure to inhaled irritants such as smoke and cat-litter dust.

Infestation with *Aleurostrongylus abstrusus*, a parasite usually known as lungworm, is thought to be fairly common in cats in the UK. Most infestations produce no symptoms and do not need treatment; a heavy infestation may cause coughing. The lifecycle of the worms involves them infesting molluscs such as slugs and snails before they can re-infest a cat who eats these creatures.

Is it serious?

Symptoms are often mild and long-term, but a cat affected by bronchial disease may suddenly develop severe breathing difficulties that require emergency treatment.

Action

If your cat starts paroxysmal coughing, leave him alone: if you handle him in any way, you may make it more difficult for him to breathe. Only move him if the room that he is in is dusty or smoky.

Close any exits from your house and monitor your cat. If he does not stop coughing in a few seconds, or his breathing is still very laboured, you should contact your vet centre immediately for further advice.

If your cat's breathing quickly settles down, treat him as normal but keep him indoors for a few days to monitor him. If he suffers from another attack, take him to your vet.

Your vet will examine your cat and listen to his breathing using a stethoscope (see page 91). He or she may stimulate your cat to cough by gently squeezing on his windpipe. Further tests may include analysis of mucus taken from the airways, blood tests, analysis of faeces to look for airway parasites, and X-ray investigations (see pages 91–2).

COMMON SYMPTOMS

The symptoms of this condition are due to airflow obstruction. This results from constriction of the lower airways because of thickening in their walls and/or a build-up of mucus and fluid.
• Typically, an affected cat will have a dry cough, which will include bouts of paroxysmal coughing.
• A severely affected cat may also be forced to breathe through his mouth rather than his nose.

Treatment

If your cat has severe breathing difficulties, your vet will give him medicines to try to open up his airways and allow him to breathe more easily. Your cat may also be given oxygen. These emergency treatments will be started before investigations are carried out. If a cause is then found, your vet will treat your cat accordingly: for instance, with wormers if your cat has lungworms, or with antibiotics if his airways are infected.

If a cause is not identified, your cat may well be suffering from an allergic reaction to something in his environment, or he may be inhaling a substance that is irritating his airways. In this case, you may need to alter his environment at home (your vet will help you to make a list of potential irritants).

It may be impossible either to identify or to remove an underlying cause of the bronchial disease from your cat's environment, and he may need treatment aimed at controlling his symptoms in the long term.

Aftercare

If possible, encourage your cat to take plenty of fresh air; inhaling steam may help to break down mucus trapped in his airways (see pages 40–1). Keep him in another room when you are vacuuming, and, if you smoke, give it up!

Exudative pleurisy (Pyothorax)

This condition is the accumulation in a cat's chest of watery pus that results from bacterial infection. This is effectively an abscess, which generally involves the whole of the inside of the chest.

Causes

The underlying cause of exudative pleurisy often remains unclear, but possibilities include the following:
• A penetrating chest wound.
• An infection under the skin: for example, from a subcutaneous abscess (see pages 60–1).
• Perforation of the oesophagus.
• Internal movement of a foreign body such as a grass awn.
• A lung infection.

Is it serious?

A cat suffering from exudative pleurisy is seriously ill, but prompt and aggressive treatment may be successful in clearing infection if it is carried out sufficiently early.

Cats at risk

All cats are at risk of this condition.

Action

If your cat exhibits any of the symptoms, take him to your vet as soon as possible. If he is having breathing difficulties, contact your vet centre immediately.

Your vet will examine your cat thoroughly, and may carry out blood tests, X-ray investigations, and analysis of a fluid sample from your cat's chest (see pages 91–2).

Treatment

If your cat has severe difficulty in breathing, your vet will need to carry out emergency procedures such as immediate chest drainage and the administration of oxygen.

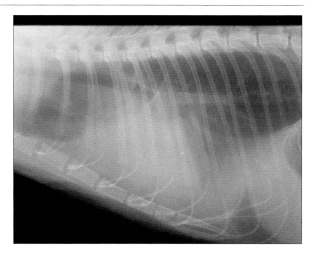

This is an X-ray picture of the chest area of a cat with exudative pleurisy. The abnormal amount of fluid within the chest and around the lungs appears white on the picture, making the heart difficult to see.

He or she will then institute a treatment regime that will have the following aims:
• To remove the underlying cause of the infection (if known).
• To drain off the pus-like fluid.
• To control the bacterial infection.
• To prevent any further formation of fluid.
Your cat will be admitted as an in-patient for this treatment. The fluid within his chest may be drawn off repeatedly using a syringe and large needle, or your vet may decide to anaesthetize him (see

pages 94–5) and insert a proper chest drain that will stay in place while he is treated with antibiotics. The drain will only be removed when the chest is free of fluid and no more is being produced. This tube may also be used to wash out your cat's chest with special antibiotic solutions.

Aftercare

When your cat returns home, you will need to continue to administer any prescribed medicines, and to nurse him back to full fitness (see pages 98–111).

Prevention

You should never ignore a bite wound suffered by your cat. Such a wound may not appear to be particularly severe at first, but may develop into an abscess that could lead to serious complications such as exudative pleurisy.

For this reason, always examine your cat thoroughly for any bite wounds if you know or think that he has been involved in a fight with another cat or with another animal (see also pages 60–1).

COMMON SYMPTOMS

In many cases, symptoms may appear to occur quite suddenly, even though the condition may have been grumbling on for some time. They are very variable, but may include any of the following:
• An increased breathing rate (the breathing rate of a normal cat is 24 to 42 breaths per minute).
• Breathing difficulty
• Dullness and depression
• Weight loss
• Fever

Feline viral upper-respiratory-tract disease

This common condition is perhaps better-known as 'cat 'flu'. It is an infectious disease that is quick to spread in situations in which many cats are kept or brought together, such as at boarding catteries and cat-rescue centres.

Causes

A number of infectious organisms may be involved in causing cat 'flu, but by far the most important of these are two viruses called feline herpesvirus (FHV), also known as feline rhinotracheitis virus, and feline calicivirus (FCV).

A cat usually becomes infected by coming into direct contact with another cat suffering from cat 'flu. However, as many cats continue to carry these viruses after they have recovered from infection, a cat may also become infected by a cat who is apparently healthy but who has had cat 'flu in the past. Contaminated objects such as feeding bowls may also be a source of infection.

Is it serious?

Cats suffering from cat 'flu can be seriously ill, but most recover. Very young or old individuals who are severely affected may die.

A cat who has recovered from this disease may go on to suffer from long-term problems such as chronic rhinitis (see pages 40–1).

Cats at risk

All cats are at risk of suffering from this condition.

Action

If your cat begins to sneeze, or shows any of the other symptoms described, you should keep him confined indoors and arrange for him to see your vet.

Your vet may be able to confirm that your cat is suffering from cat 'flu just by examining him, but he or she may not be able to tell which of the two main viruses is involved. If it is necessary to find this out, he or she will take a swab from your cat's throat for analysis.

Treatment

There are currently no anti-viral medicines in general use, but prompt treatment is still essential to prevent short- and long-term complications. Treatment is based on nursing to encourage an affected cat to continue to eat and drink (see pages 104–5), and on medicines to alleviate symptoms. Your cat may require any or all of the following:

Antibiotics • These may be given to control bacterial infections, which may occur as a result of tissue damage caused by the initial viral infection.

Mucolytics • These medicines may be used to help to break down and to clear the mucus build-up in your cat's respiratory system.

Multi-vitamin preparations • These may be prescribed to stimulate your cat's appetite.

Special fluids • These may be given via an intravenous drip (see page 93) if your cat's illness has made him dehydrated and he is not drinking.

Liquid food • This may need to be force-fed through a special feeding tube if your cat will not eat (see pages 104–5).

Aftercare

If your cat is seriously ill, he may need to be admitted as an in-patient at his vet centre for intensive care.

However, if you are willing and able to nurse your cat at home, your vet may ask you to do so, as your cat will be happier at home and will also be more likely to eat. Your vet will advise you of all that you need to do for your cat. This may include cleaning away any discharge from

COMMON SYMPTOMS

The precise symptoms shown will vary depending on the cause, and on the cat's immune system's ability to cope with the infection. FHV often causes severe symptoms; FCV may not result in any symptoms at all or may result in similar symptoms to those of FHV, depending on the viral strain involved. The following are all typical symptoms of cat 'flu:
• Reluctance to eat, and depression.
• Fever
• Sneezing
• Reddened, inflamed eyes
• Nasal discharge
• Coughing (occasionally)
• Tongue ulcers (especially with feline calicivirus infection).

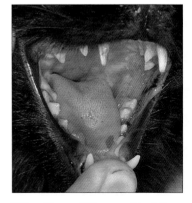

This cat has cat 'flu caused by feline herpesvirus: one of the symptoms is the red, inflamed ulcer on his tongue.

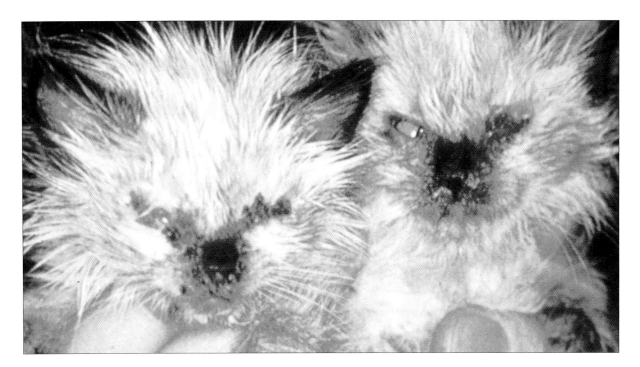

These two cats are showing typical symptoms associated with cat 'flu, including a mucky discharge from the eyes and nose.

his eyes and nose, keeping him warm (he must stay indoors) and encouraging him to eat and drink, as well as carrying out general nursing duties (see pages 98–111).

It may take several weeks for your cat to recover from the initial infection. Once he has suffered from cat 'flu, you must also assume that he is a carrier of the virus.

Eight out of 10 cats infected with feline herpesvirus become lifelong carriers. However, if your cat were infected by this virus, he is only likely to be infectious to other cats intermittently – especially if he becomes stressed either mentally or physically (for example, by moving house or by suffering from another infectious disease).

At these times, your cat will shed the 'flu virus into the environment, even though he may not exhibit any symptoms himself. If he was infected by feline calicivirus, he is very likely to shed viruses into the environment continually for a short

time, although he may do so for up to two years (if you do not know the virus with which your cat was infected, you should assume that either may have been involved).

You must try to ensure that, after recovering from cat 'flu, your cat leads as stress-free a life as possible. If a female cat has suffered from cat 'flu in the past and is now pregnant, ask your vet for specific advice.

Prevention

Vaccination improves the speed and effectiveness of a cat's immune response to infection by stimulating it through exposure to an organism before the cat meets it for real. You must make sure that your cat is regularly and routinely vaccinated against both feline herpesvirus and feline calicivirus.

These vaccines may not actually prevent your cat from becoming infected or lessen the chance of him becoming a virus carrier after his recovery, but they will significantly

reduce the severity of the disease should he become infected. They are normally combined with other vaccinations as part of a typical regime (see page 85). This usually involves two doses three to four weeks apart, followed by 'booster' doses at 12-month intervals.

Newborn kittens receive some natural protection against these viruses from their mothers, but this is shortlived. In most cases, they should receive their primary-vaccination course when they are between nine and 12 weeks old.

Even a cat who has suffered from cat 'flu should be vaccinated on a regular basis. This is because his natural immunity resulting from real infection is shortlived, and because there are many strains of FCV that may cause the disease.

Chronic rhinitis

Sometimes colloquially known as 'chronic snuffles', chronic rhinitis is a longstanding inflammatory condition that affects the internal lining of a cat's nose.

Causes

Cases of chronic rhinitis occur most commonly as a follow-on to feline viral upper-respiratory-tract disease (see pages 38–9).

Is it serious?

Controlling the symptoms of this condition can be difficult, and an affected cat may require very long-term treatment.

Some cats who are suffering from chronic rhinitis may be long-term carriers of feline herpesvirus (FHV) and feline calicivirus (FCV), the viruses responsible for cat 'flu, and so may present a risk to other cats with whom they have contact.

Cats at risk

All unvaccinated cats are at risk of suffering from cat 'flu, the main underlying cause of chronic rhinitis.

Action

If your cat begins to sneeze and he has a nasal discharge, you should contact your vet centre as soon as possible. This is because, if he has cat 'flu, prompt and appropriate treatment should help to limit the degree of damage that is caused to the internal lining of his nose.

You must keep your cat indoors while he is ill. This is not only so that he will stay warm and rested, and so that you can monitor his progress, but also because he may be infectious to other cats.

If your cat sneezes occasionally and has a longstanding nasal discharge – either from the time

COMMON SYMPTOMS

Most cats with chronic rhinitis remain in generally good health. However, common symptoms include the following:
• A yellow, grey or green mucus discharge from the nostrils for at least four weeks.
• Occasional sneezing
• Occasional lack of appetite

that you first collected him as a kitten or following an episode of cat 'flu since he has been living with you – you should arrange for him to be examined at your vet centre. Do not ignore the symptoms of chronic rhinitis. They are very unlikely to resolve naturally, and, the longer your cat is left untreated, the more difficult his symptoms may be to bring under control.

Your vet will consider the history of your cat's symptoms carefully. He or she will then examine your cat thoroughly, and may wish to carry out any or all of the following:
• X-ray investigations of your cat's nose and sinuses (see page 91)
• Laboratory analysis of a sample of any nasal discharge (see page 92)
• Specific blood tests: for instance, to look for evidence of an existing feline leukaemia virus or feline immunodeficiency virus infection (see pages 80–3), as either or both of these could be adversely affecting your cat's immune response to the infection in his nose.

Treatment

The management of chronic rhinitis in a cat can be very difficult. This is because, once there is permanent damage to the lining of the nose, the normally harmless bacteria that

---

ALLOWING YOUR CAT OUTDOORS

If your cat has chronic rhinitis, or bronchial disease (see page 36), ensuring that he spends time in a fresh-air environment may help to ease his symptoms.

If you are unwilling or unable to give your cat free access outdoors, alternatives are to fence off your garden or to build a totally enclosed outdoor cage. The following are all important points to consider.

FENCING OFF YOUR GARDEN
• An adult cat can clamber through a hole in a fence just 10 cm (4 in) wide, so check carefully around the perimeter of your garden.
• Any boundary structure should be at least 3 m (10 ft) high with wire-mesh fencing angled inwards on top with a narrow net 'roof' attached.

• Trees with branches that overhang the fence may provide a high-rise walkway out of your garden, so prune back any that your cat could use as a ladder or bridge.
• Gates are an obvious escape route. Double gates are preferable, so that one can be closed before the next is opened.

AN OUTDOOR ENCLOSURE
A number of companies build cat runs to order, or you could build one yourself. This should contain the following as a minimum:
• A weather-proof cabin or den
• A covered toileting area, housing a litter-tray
• Shelves or perches
• Entertainment, such as branches to climb and a variety of toys

live in that part of the body can cause problems in a cat at almost any time. However, treatment may include the following.

Antibiotics • Your vet is likely to prescribe appropriate antibiotics for administration by mouth (see pages 101–2) for an initial period of four to six weeks. In many cases the symptoms soon return when antibiotics are stopped, so your cat may need to be given repeated courses of antibiotics as and when necessary.

Other medicines • Your vet may also prescribe medicines called mucolytics to help to clear the congestion in your cat's nose.

Surgery • An operation to remove diseased tissue and to flush out affected sinuses is normally only considered in the worst cases, as results are often disappointing.

Steam inhalation can help a great deal in clearing the nasal congestion suffered by a cat with chronic rhinitis. Keep a close eye on your cat during this procedure to ensure that he remains calm and comfortable.

Aftercare

At home, you will need to keep your cat's nose and face clean, and to administer his medicines (see pages 101–2). You may also need to encourage him to eat, as he is likely to have a reduced sense of smell.

Steam inhalation may help to clear your cat's nasal congestion, so encourage him to stay in your bathroom when you are having a bath or a shower. Alternatively, a better option will be to put him into his carrying basket and to place a bowl of steaming-hot water near it. Cover the basket and the bowl with a towel, so that your cat has to inhale the steam. Adding a few drops of a decongestant such as menthol or eucalyptus to the water (you should be able to obtain these from your local pharmacy) may

also help. Watch your cat during this procedure to make sure that he does not become distressed.

Although some cats with chronic rhinitis seem to improve if they are kept outdoors, this may not be a suitable or acceptable management option for you or your cat. Before altering your cat's normal routine, it will be a good idea to discuss your plans either with your vet or with a veterinary nurse.

Prevention

You must ensure that your cat is routinely vaccinated against the major viruses that cause upper-respiratory-tract disease, or cat 'flu (see pages 38–9).

The prompt treatment of a cat who is suffering from cat 'flu will lessen the likelihood of him going on to suffer from chronic rhinitis.

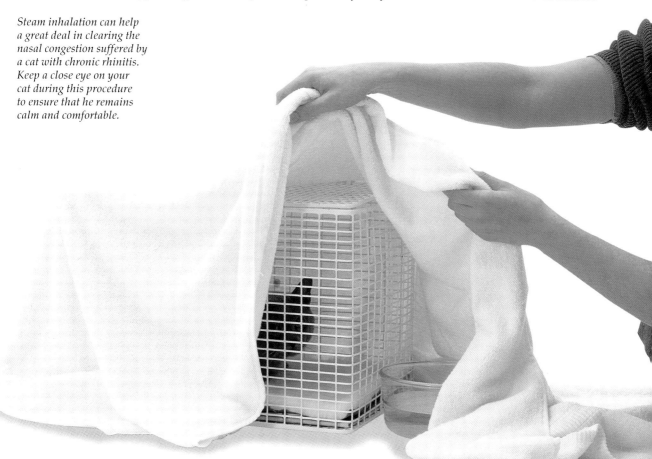

Joints, ligaments and bones

Most cats are naturally extremely agile and athletic animals, but inevitably their joints, ligaments and bones are vulnerable to accidental damage, and to the wear and tear of everyday life. However, thanks to their lightness, sense of balance, ability to land on their feet and built-in shock-absorbers (their forelegs are not connected by bone to the rest of the skeleton), cats do not suffer from as many orthopaedic problems as they might otherwise do. These conditions in cats occur most commonly as a result of road accidents.

Arthritis

Cats can suffer from different kinds of arthritis, which literally means 'joint inflammation'. However, arthritis is much more complex than simple inflammation, so this name is rather misleading.

For instance, osteoarthritis is associated with the growth of new bone around a moveable joint and the deterioration of the smooth cartilage that covers and protects the ends of the bones within it; the tissues that line the joint may not necessarily be inflamed.

Causes

The following forms of arthritis are most commonly suffered by cats.

Traumatic arthritis ('sprain') • This may be caused by sudden injury to a joint: for instance, following impact with a moving vehicle, as the result of a fight with another cat or due to an awkward fall. The injury to the joint may include tearing or stretching of the soft tissues and ligaments within and surrounding the joint. The bones within it or their cartilage coverings may also be damaged.

Osteoarthritis • This is considered by experts to be the end result of a joint failure that may occur for any reason. The shoulder and elbow joints are those most frequently affected in older cats. Common causes are recurrent episodes of traumatic arthritis (possibly due to a cat's athletic lifestyle), and also dislocations of joints or fractures involving joints (see pages 44–6) that occurred in the past and made the joints more susceptible to excessive wear and tear.

Is it serious?

Traumatic arthritis in a joint that results from a minor sprain is likely to be painful for a short time but is not serious. However, the damage inflicted through impact with a vehicle may be much more severe, and may involve fractures to the bones within the joint that require surgery (see pages 45–7).

The seriousness of osteoarthritis depends on the nature and severity of any underlying cause, on the joints affected and on the general health status of the cat involved. A cat who is overweight will always suffer more than one who is not obese (see pages 76–7).

Arthritis is a painful condition, and for this reason it should always be taken seriously.

Cats at risk

Any type of cat may suffer from arthritis. However, it is a condition that is perhaps most common in cats who lead athletic lives.

Action

If your cat suddenly begins to limp badly, you should take appropriate action (see page 47).

If your cat limps intermittently, is regularly stiff after rest, or is less athletic and agile than formerly, take him to see your vet. Do not wait until your cat is hobbling about: if he has osteoarthritis, the

COMMON SYMPTOMS

Symptoms of traumatic arthritis may include the following:
• A swollen joint
• A painful joint, causing limping on that leg and resentment of the joint being handled.

Symptoms of osteoarthritis may include the following:
• Limping or stiffness: this may be mild or intermittent initially, but will gradually become worse over time. Typically, any lameness or stiffness may be more pronounced after rest, and may appear to wear off when the cat has been moving about for a few minutes. The stiffness shown by an affected cat may also become worse in cold and damp weather.
• An abnormal appearance to a joint, due to the new bone formation around it.
• Sudden and more severe lameness may occur if a joint that is affected by osteoarthritis is suddenly sprained.

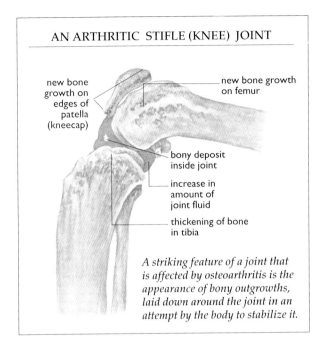

AN ARTHRITIC STIFLE (KNEE) JOINT

new bone growth on edges of patella (kneecap)

new bone growth on femur

bony deposit inside joint

increase in amount of joint fluid

thickening of bone in tibia

A striking feature of a joint that is affected by osteoarthritis is the appearance of bony outgrowths, laid down around the joint in an attempt by the body to stabilize it.

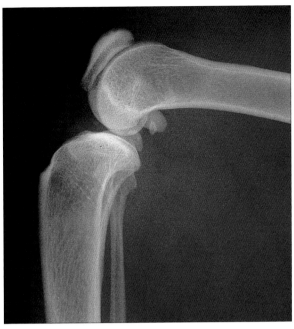

sooner you know, the sooner you will be able to adopt measures to slow down its progression.

Your vet will consider your cat's symptoms, and will examine him thoroughly both at rest and while he is moving about. He or she will also need to manipulate your cat's joints in order to identify whether they are painful.

Once your vet has identified which joint (or joints) is affected, he or she may carry out further tests, including X-ray investigations and possibly analysis of fluid taken from the joints (see pages 91–2).

Treatment

This will depend on the cause and severity of the arthritis. A sudden, uncomplicated case of traumatic arthritis – such as a simple sprain – will usually respond well to strict rest for a few days and to a short course of anti-inflammatory medicines; a more severe case of traumatic arthritis may require supportive dressings.

The treatment of a cat suffering from established osteoarthritis is likely to include the following:

Anti-inflammatory medicines • Ideally, these should only be used in the short term, as and when necessary to encourage movement. You must not think of them as miracle cures simply because your cat's stiffness disappears when he is on them. In most cases these medicines are acting simply as painkillers, and should only be used in addition to weight control and good exercise management.

Dietary management • Weight control is an important feature of any treatment for arthritis. If your cat is overweight, you must follow the dietary advice of your vet (see also pages 76–7).

Exercise management • Although it is very difficult to impose an exercise regime on a cat, those individuals who are affected by osteoarthritis will benefit from regular activity. A small amount

This is an X-ray picture of a normal, healthy stifle joint. Note the rounded surfaces at the bone edges: these would be roughened in an osteoarthritic joint.

of exercise taken frequently is recommended, so be prepared to wake up your cat for a wander about every now and again, and avoid letting him sleep in one place for hours at a time.

Surgery • This may be appropriate for osteoarthritis. (Some cases of traumatic arthritis may also need surgical treatment.)

As osteoarthritis is a progressive condition, the treatment in any given case will need to be adapted from time to time.

Aftercare

Keeping your cat's joints (and the rest of his body) warm will help, as may massage of his joints and physiotherapy: ask your vet or a veterinary nurse for advice on the techniques to use, as well as for a practical demonstration.

Joint dislocation

A dislocation (or luxation, as it is also called) occurs when the ends of two or more bones that normally articulate together in a joint become permanently separated. The joints most commonly dislocated by cats include the hip, the stifle (or knee), the carpus (or wrist), the tarsus (or ankle) and the jaw.

Causes

Almost all dislocations suffered by cats occur as a result of traumatic injury. An injury of this kind may occur if a cat is involved in a road-traffic accident, for example, or if he jumps down or falls from a great height and lands awkwardly.

Is it serious?

If a joint dislocation is not treated promptly, a cat may suffer from pain and disability in the long term.

Cats at risk

All cats are at risk of suffering from a joint dislocation, but those cats who have a very athletic lifestyle will obviously be especially prone to an injury of this kind.

Action

If your cat is involved in any kind of accident, or you think that he may have been, you should contact your vet centre immediately – even if your cat does not appear to be very badly injured.

Your vet will examine your cat thoroughly to confirm the nature and extent of any injuries that are associated with his symptoms, and also to check that he does not have any other, less obvious but possibly more serious, injuries. Expect your vet to advise that a thorough X-ray investigation is carried out on your cat (see also page 91).

COMMON SYMPTOMS

The precise symptoms will depend on the joint involved and also on any other injuries sustained. For example, tendons and ligaments, as well as other supporting structures such as muscles, may have been damaged when the bones separated. Other symptoms may include the following:
• With a dislocated limb joint, a cat is unlikely to be able to bear weight normally on that limb (see page 47).
• A jaw that is dislocated will make it impossible for a cat to close his mouth properly.
• A dislocated joint will often be one of several injuries (even if these are only skin cuts). For instance, a cat with a dislocated jaw may well have a bleeding mouth or nose, and may have missing or damaged teeth.
• Many cats are somehow able to struggle home, even after having been fairly seriously injured in an accident. You may come home to find your cat resting and think nothing of this – it may only be at some point later on, when you realize that he has not moved, that you become aware that something is wrong.
• A telltale sign that a cat has been involved in a road-traffic accident is frayed claws (see page 63).

Treatment

A joint dislocation is not normally life-threatening, so your vet may delay treatment for this if your cat has other more serious problems that require immediate attention.

For a hip • Having anaesthetized your cat (see pages 94–5), your vet will try to put the ball at the end of the femur, or thigh bone, back into its corresponding socket in the pelvis. Your cat will need strict rest for about four weeks after this, for the first week of which he should be confined (see page 106). If during his convalescence or soon after returning to normal activity your cat dislocates his hip again, your vet may decide to operate to pin the joint together, or to remove the ball from the end of the femur. A 'false' joint between the end of the femur and the pelvis will then form.

For a stifle, carpus or tarsus • A dislocation involving any of these joints will normally be treated surgically. Your vet is likely to insert metal pins in order to fix the bones into their normal positions.

For a jaw • One or both 'hinge' joints of the jaw on either side of the face may become dislocated. With your cat anaesthetized (see pages 94–5), your vet will place a small rod across the back of his mouth to act as a fulcrum, against which the lower jaw can be levered back into place.

Aftercare

At home, your cat will need special care during convalescence from the dislocation and any other injuries (see pages 98–111). You must keep him indoors until he has recovered, and to ensure that he rests you may have to restrict him to a cage at first (see page 106).

You must take your cat to your vet centre for check-ups: these may involve further X-ray investigations (see page 91) to assess the rate of healing of the dislocated joint, and surgery to remove any metal pins inserted as part of the treatment.

Bone fracture

A bone is described as fractured when it has cracked, split, bent, shattered or snapped into two or more pieces. A so-called simple, or closed, fracture is one in which the overlying skin remains intact. In a compound, or open, fracture there is some kind of hole through the skin, in the form of a wound, that leads down to where the bone or bones are damaged.

Although, due to the athletic lifestyle of many cats, the bones of the legs and feet are perhaps most commonly affected, any bone in a cat's body may fracture, including those of the skull, jaw, rib cage, spine, shoulder blades and pelvis.

Causes

The majority of fractures are caused by direct injury to a bone or bones as a result of road-traffic accidents or bad falls.

Other possible causes of bone fractures include being trodden on or kicked by another animal, excessive muscle contractions or gunshot injuries. Even everyday movements may be sufficient to fracture bones that have been weakened by another condition, such as cancer (see pages 68–9).

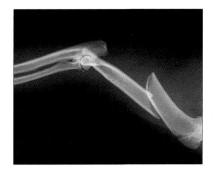

This is an X-ray picture of a simple complete fracture of the humerus bone of a two-year-old cat.

Is it serious?

Bone- (orthopaedic-) surgery techniques used on cats are very advanced (see page 46). As a result, most fractures can be repaired, although a cat may be permanently disabled to some extent due to the severity of his injuries.

In a severe accident, a fracture may be one of several injuries to other body parts, such as major organs, blood vessels and nerves.

Cats at risk

All cats are at risk of suffering from a bone fracture, especially if they roam near busy roads or lead very

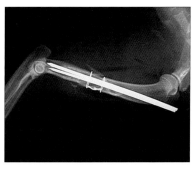

To repair the fracture, metal pins were inserted into the cavity, and wire bands were used to hold the bone fragments.

athletic lives. Individuals who have weak bones – such as very young kittens, or cats suffering from other bone diseases such as cancer (see pages 68–9) – may be more at risk than healthy adult cats.

Action

If your cat has been involved in an accident of any kind, contact your vet centre immediately so that he can be checked over, even if he does not appear at first sight to be seriously injured.

You should deal with any of the symptoms associated with a bone fracture as emergencies until they are proven otherwise by your vet, and you may need to carry out appropriate first-aid procedures (see pages 114–17).

Your vet will examine your cat thoroughly, as well as carrying out X-ray investigations (see page 91).

If your cat has severe multiple injuries, your vet will initially concentrate on keeping him alive, and may therefore only undertake immediate repairs to any fractures considered to be life-threatening. He or she may simply stabilize any less-serious fractures temporarily,

---

COMMON SYMPTOMS

The symptoms associated with this condition will depend on the number and type of bones affected, the type of fracture(s) involved and the cause. They may include the following:
• Obvious skin wounds (the broken bone ends may be visible).
• Marked swelling of the tissues surrounding the fracture.
• Unusual behaviour as a result of pain, such as unexpected aggression

when handled (a cat who is in severe pain may also purr continuously).
• An abnormal appearance or outline associated with the affected part of the body.
• Inability to use the affected body part: a broken leg may be held off the ground; a major fracture of the spine or pelvis may cause paraplegia; a fracture in more than one leg will make it impossible for a cat to stand.

COMMON TYPES OF FRACTURE

In a simple fracture the skin is intact, whereas in a compound fracture the bone is exposed. In a complete fracture the bone has separated, while a comminuted fracture has several pieces.

simple
complete fracture

compound
complete fracture

simple, complete
comminuted fracture

using splints or other dressings, or may restrict your cat to a small cage to prevent him from moving. Attempts at repairing these bones can then be carried out when your cat is in a more stable condition.

Your vet should give painkillers to your cat to make him feel more comfortable, and may treat him with antibiotics if necessary.

Treatment

A fractured bone will repair itself, provided that the broken ends are held in the correct positions while natural healing takes place. The aim of treatment is to put the broken pieces into their normal anatomical relationship and to prevent them from moving. The more closely the broken ends are held together, the sooner the bone will repair itself.

The following are all commonly employed techniques:

External manipulation • This will be carried out to put the broken bone ends back into a normal alignment, and will be followed by the application of a rigid cast or splint to prevent the pieces from moving. This technique is normally only appropriate in certain kinds of 'simple' fracture in the bones of the legs and feet.

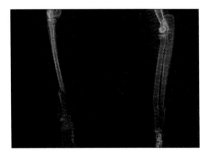

This X-ray of a cat's foreleg shows a simple complete fracture of both bones that join the elbow to the wrist (carpus). The picture on the left is a front view; the one on the right a side view.

Insertion of a metal pin • In this surgical procedure, a pin (or pins) is inserted into the marrow cavity of a broken bone, to keep the two largest pieces in position. Wires may be tightened around the bone, to prevent movement of the main pieces and to attach any smaller bone fragments.

Fixing fragments of bone • Bone fragments may be fixed back into position using special screws.

Metal plates • These may be screwed to two or more pieces of bone to hold them together.

Fine pins through the skin • Bone fragments may be held rigidly in position by passing fine pins into them through the skin. These are inserted in carefully chosen positions, then bolted together on the outside to make a strong, supporting metal 'scaffold' (when the bone has healed, this will be removed).

Rather than being treated surgically, certain fractures – such as some types involving the pelvis – may be left alone if your vet considers that surgery may cause your cat more problems than it will solve. Such cats are normally restricted in a small cage for several weeks, to enforce rest while natural healing is given a chance to take place.

The speed at which a fracture heals will depend on the age of the cat (in a young cat, a broken bone may be completely back to normal in six weeks; in an older cat, this may take four months), and on how close together and how rigidly fixed the healing bone edges are. Bones broken into just two pieces usually heal faster than those broken into many fragments. The presence of infection will delay healing.

Aftercare

Depending on the severity of the fracture and your cat's condition, he may stay at your vet centre just for the day of his operation, or for several days or even weeks.

When he returns home, you must administer his medicines (see pages 101–2), keep any dressings clean and dry (see pages 108–9), and follow your vet's instructions regarding his exercise management.

You must also take him back to your vet centre for further X-rays to check how the fracture is healing.

Any internal metalwork may be left permanently in place, but your vet may remove any pins, screws, plates or wires if they could cause your cat problems later on.

Lameness

A cat is described as being lame if he appears to be unable to move, or if he cannot bear weight normally on one or more of his legs.

Causes

Rather than being a condition in its own right, lameness is a symptom of other underlying conditions, most of them painful. These include foreign bodies – such as thorns or grass seeds – becoming stuck in one of his paws, cuts or other wounds such as those caused during fights with another cat, arthritis (see pages 42–3), bone fractures (see pages 45–6), cat-bite wounds and abscesses (see pages 60–1), claw conditions (see page 63) and nerve disorders that may affect sensation in a leg or muscle control.

Action

If your cat is suddenly severely lame and will not bear any weight on his affected leg, put him in his carrying basket so that he will remain warm, quiet and rested while you contact your vet centre (see also page 117).

If your cat is limping a little, try to identify which leg (or legs) is causing the problem. In most cases of sudden-onset lameness, only one

COMMON SYMPTOMS

These will depend on the severity of the problem and your cat's personality, but may include:
• Reluctance to bear any weight on the affected leg.
• A hobbling gait
• An abnormal appearance to the affected leg.
• Resentment of handling
• Excessive grooming of the leg

REMOVING A FOREIGN BODY FROM YOUR CAT'S PAW

Ask someone else to restrain your cat properly (see pages 98–100), then gently try to pull out the foreign body using a suitable pair of tweezers. If you succeed in doing so, bathe the affected paw in warm, salty water for a few minutes, then bathe it with an veterinary antiseptic solution, before drying the paw gently but thoroughly.

Keep your cat indoors for a few days, and check his paw frequently. If it begins to swell, if your cat grooms it excessively or if he remains lame, contact your vet centre.

leg is affected. If the offending limb is not immediately obvious, watch your cat move about (shut his cat flap beforehand so that he cannot leave your house).

A subtle lameness involving a foreleg is easiest to pinpoint if you try to spot which foreleg your cat lunges on to when he walks: this will be his good leg. He will appear to drop his shoulder on this leg as he tries to shift his weight away from the one that is painful.

Once you have identified the problem leg, you should examine every part of it systematically, starting with your cat's claws (see also page 63). To protect yourself from being bitten or scratched, ask someone to help you to handle your cat while you examine him (see pages 98–9). Your aim will be to identify the precise part (or parts) of the leg that hurts your cat. You should know when you discover a painful area by his reaction.

If you are in any doubt as to whether your cat's response to being touched in a particular place is significant, examine the same area on his other leg and see how he responds. If he reacts in the same way with this leg, his earlier response is probably not relevant.

Examine any painful area in greater detail, and look out for the following signs:

A foreign body • If you locate a foreign body – such as a thorn – you may be able to remove it (see above).

A cut or other wound • Look for cat-bite puncture wounds (see pages 60–1). Deal with any other wounds using appropriate first-aid techniques (see page 118).

A painful or swollen joint • Apply a cold compress, such as a cloth dampened with very cold water, to control the swelling.

If you are unable to find an obvious cause of your cat's lameness, but his symptoms are not severe, force him to rest for 24 hours (see page 106) and reassess the situation. If he is still lame, contact your vet centre.

If you have been able to identify the cause, but the lameness has not improved despite first aid and 24 hours' rest, arrange for your vet to examine him. If the lameness has improved to some extent, keep your cat indoors until he is completely sound on the leg.

Your vet will examine your cat to confirm the lame leg, and will look at it in detail. He or she may carry out joint manipulations, as well as X-ray investigations (see page 91). Nerve tests may also be required.

Treatment

The precise treatment will depend on the cause of the lameness.

Skin and coat

Problems with the skin and coat are perhaps the most common reason for cats in the UK being taken to their vet centres. If your cat suffers from a condition of this kind, it is very important that his symptoms are fully investigated in a thorough attempt to identify the underlying cause or causes. It is often very easy to use drugs to control certain major symptoms – such as scratching – but unless the cause is found and specific treatment given (where possible), the symptoms will soon recur once the drugs are stopped.

Alopecia

Alopecia is a complete or a partial lack of hair in areas in which hair is normally present. It is a symptom of a number of underlying conditions.

Causes

An individual who is suffering from an infestation of skin parasites (see pages 54–8), a hypersensitivity reaction (see pages 52–3) or any other 'itchy' condition may develop areas of baldness through excessive nibbling, grooming and scratching to relieve the irritation.

Friction created by a collar may cause a bald ring to form around a cat's neck underneath it.

Dermatophytosis, a fungal skin condition commonly referred to as 'ringworm' (see opposite), may cause alopecia, as may moulting abnormalities: for instance, many hairs may be lost at the same time due to pregnancy, lactation or as a reaction to some drugs.

Stress may cause some cats to groom themselves excessively. The resulting hair-thinning is referred to as psychogenic alopecia, and seems to be found most commonly in the Siamese, Burmese, Himalayan and Abyssinian breeds.

The precise causes of some types of alopecia remain unknown. An example of this is that, every so often, some Siamese cats lose the fur on their ear flaps in a condition known as pinnal alopecia (the fur regrows spontaneously after several months). The cause (or causes) of feline symmetric alopecia – perhaps the most dramatic type of alopecia to be suffered by cats (see below, left) – is not fully understood.

Although it is a completely unnatural condition, alopecia in some breeds of cat – such as the hairless sphynx – is considered normal by some cat authorities.

Is it serious?

Alopecia may be associated with serious underlying conditions such as hypersensitivity reactions (see pages 52–3), so all cases of baldness should be taken seriously until they are proved otherwise by a vet.

A cat who is suffering from feline symmetric alopecia may not look his best, but he is likely to be very happy and healthy in every other respect.

Cats at risk

The risk depends on the cause of this condition.

Action

If you spot an obvious bald patch on your cat, or he develops a sparse coat, take him to see your vet. If he is scratching and grooming himself excessively, you should take him as

---

COMMON SYMPTOMS

The areas of the coat affected by alopecia will depend on its cause.
• A cat suffering from an 'itchy' condition will normally develop alopecia of the parts of his body that he can scratch, lick, nibble or rub.
• Affected areas may contain broken hairs, and the skin may be inflamed and scabby/crusty.
• In alopecia that has resulted from moulting abnormalities, large areas of the coat may be involved.
• Feline symmetric alopecia may cause severe hair thinning of the abdomen, of the inner and outer thighs and backs of the hindlegs, of the forelegs from elbow to wrist, around the anus and genitals, under the chest and in the armpits.

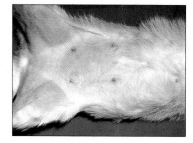

This cat has a type of alopecia called telogen defluxion, in which many hairs have moulted simultaneously.

(Note: thinning of the hair-coat over the temples, between the eyes and ears, is normal in cats. It is especially noticeable in short-haired types.)

soon you can, to prevent him from damaging his skin unnecessarily.

Your vet will consider your cat's symptoms, and will examine him thoroughly. He or she may also carry out a number of other tests and procedures: these may include blood tests, examination of skin and hair samples to look for parasites (see pages 54–8) and to decide whether hairs are being broken by excessive grooming or are being shed, and intradermal skin tests (see page 53). Attempts may also be made to culture the fungus that causes dermatophytosis.

Treatment

Many of the underlying causes of alopecia in cats are treatable with appropriate medicines. Pinnal alopecia does not require treatment; psychogenic alopecia may respond to behavioural therapy.

The hair loss associated with feline symmetric alopecia may be reversed by the use of drugs such as thyroid hormones or certain sex-hormone preparations. However, such therapies carry the risk of severe side-effects in the long term, so some cases are left untreated.

NORMAL MOULTING

• Each hair grows to a set length governed by a cat's genes. After a variable period, the hair is shed.
• A cat does not go bald when shedding his coat, or moulting, because no two hairs near each other are at the same part of the growth cycle at the same time.
• Most cats have periods of heavy coat replacement, or moulting, in the spring and summer. At these times, some cats may grow over 1 km (⅔ mile) of hair a day!

Dermatophytosis

Dermatophytosis is a condition caused by infection of hair, claws or the dead outer layers of skin by certain types of fungus. It is more often referred to as 'ringworm'.

Causes

Dermatophytosis may be caused by one of three fungi: *Microsporum canis*, *Microsporum gypseum* and *Trichophyton mentagrophytes*. Almost all cases in the UK are caused by *Microsporum canis*. A cat becomes infected by contact with an infected animal or with a contaminated object such as a brush or bedding.

COMMON SYMPTOMS

• Lesions caused by this fungus are most common on the head, ear flaps and paws, and are typically in the form of single or multiple, circular or irregularly shaped areas of alopecia: these areas may contain broken hairs and dandruff. The lesions are rarely itchy. (Note: some long- and fine-haired cats may carry ringworm without showing any symptoms.)

Is it serious?

An affected cat may self-cure in one to six months, but ringworm should be taken seriously as it also affects people (see right).

Cats at risk

Any cat may suffer from ringworm, although young and long-haired cats – especially of the Persian and Himalayan breeds – seem more prone to it. Ringworm may be more common in hot, humid climates.

Action

If you notice any typical lesions on your cat's skin, you should take him to your vet.

Your vet will examine your cat thoroughly. He or she may also carry out microscopic examinations of hair samples, and may look at your cat's fur in ultraviolet light (in about 50 per cent of cases involving *Microsporum canis*, affected hairs and skin scabs will fluoresce bright green in this light). An attempt may also be made in the laboratory to culture the fungus from samples of hair and skin debris.

ZOONOSIS

Approximately 50 per cent of all people who come into contact with a cat who has ringworm are likely to catch it themselves. If your cat is diagnosed as suffering from ringworm, and you or any member of your family have any skin lesions, inform your doctor.

Treatment

Ringworm may be a self-limiting condition, but most affected cats are treated. The treatment regime will depend on the nature of the lesions, but may include the following:
• Clipping the hair from all lesions
• Topical treatment of lesions
• The administration of anti-fungal medicine in food (see page 101), except to pregnant queens. This must be continued for two weeks after an apparent cure is achieved.
• Ringworm can survive in the environment for over four years, so any items – such as bedding – that may be contaminated must be destroyed and, where possible, the cat's environment disinfected.

Eosinophilic granuloma complex

Eosinophilic granuloma complex is not a specific disease or condition in its own right, but refers to a group of three different types of skin lesion that are suffered by some cats. These are called eosinophilic or 'rodent' ulcers, eosinophilic plaque and eosinophilic granuloma. An affected cat may have more than one type of lesion at the same time.

Causes

The three types of lesions are most commonly suffered by those cats who already have existing skin hypersensitivities (see pages 52–3). Bacterial infection may also make the symptoms worse.

In some cases, susceptibility to these lesions is thought to be passed from one generation to the next, but the precise cause is often unknown.

Is it serious?

An unresolved eosinophilic ulcer may become cancerous.

Cats at risk

All three types of lesion occur more commonly in female cats.

The 'scooped-out', glistening area on this cat's upper lip is an eosinophilic ulcer (also known as a 'rodent' ulcer).

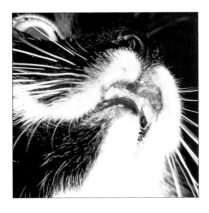

COMMON SYMPTOMS

• Most eosinophilic ulcers occur on one side of the upper lip, although they may also appear in an affected cat's mouth or on other areas of his skin. The ulcers are red-brown in colour, hairless, and have a raised edge and a glistening appearance.
• Eosinophilic plaque lesions are normally found on the abdomen or inner thighs. They are typically round or oval, red, moist, raised areas of tissue that are intensely itchy.
• Most eosinophilic granuloma lesions occur on the backs of the thighs, in the mouth and on the face. On the thighs they appear typically as a line of raised, firm yellow or pink tissue. These lesions are one of the most common reasons for lower lip swellings and nodules on cats.

Action

If your cat starts to show any of the symptoms described, you should arrange for him to be examined by your vet as soon as possible.

Your vet will probably be able to confirm that your cat is suffering from eosinophilic granuloma complex simply by examining the lesions on his skin. Depending on the outcome of this examination, he or she may then wish to carry out additional procedures to identify any underlying conditions, particularly hypersensitivity reactions that may need specific treatment (see pages 52–3).

Microscopic examination of a biopsy (see page 92) taken from a longstanding eosinophilic ulcer will help to determine whether the ulcer has become cancerous.

Treatment

The precise treatment regime that your vet adopts will depend on the type and extent of the lesions, and on any underlying conditions that have been identified. In most cases, medical treatment is carried out using steroids administered by injection and/or mouth, or using other anti-inflammatory medicines given by mouth (see page 97). Your vet will prescribe antibiotics if he or she thinks that bacterial infection is complicating the condition.

An eosinophilic ulcer that fails to respond well to medical therapy may need to be surgically cut away. Alternative approaches to this type of ulcer include the following:
• Radiotherapy (see page 69)
• Laser therapy
• Surgical removal of the ulcer
• Cryosurgery: a technique that involves the repeated freezing and thawing of diseased tissue.

Aftercare

At home, you will need to nurse your cat and attend to his lesions as you have been instructed by your vet or veterinary nurse.

If your vet has prescribed a course of medicines for your cat, you will need to continue their administration (see pages 101–2). This treatment may need to be continued for several weeks.

Eosinophilic plaque is a very itchy condition, so your cat may need to wear an 'Elizabethan collar' at first (see page 108) to prevent him from making his lesions worse while drug treatments take effect. You should also keep him confined indoors until he has fully recovered.

Fur mats

Many pet cats, such as Persians, have fashionable – but unnatural – coats that we have helped to create through selective breeding. It is almost impossible for these cats to look after their coats properly, and so their fur is prone to matting.

A fur mat usually forms from loose hairs that have not been shed or removed from the coat, and have become tangled together with hairs still firmly embedded in the skin.

Causes

The most common cause of matted fur is inadequate grooming.

Is it serious?

A tangled and matted coat does not insulate a cat's body effectively, and fails to protect the underlying skin from damage.

An affected cat may find a mat in his coat uncomfortable, and may damage his own skin by trying to groom it out. A mat may also affect the temperature and humidity at the skin surface, making it prone to inflammation and infection.

Cats at risk

The cats most at risk of fur mats are those belonging to owners who do not groom them regularly enough.

COMMON SYMPTOMS

A mat is easy to feel. It may form anywhere on a cat's body, but the most common sites are as follows:
• Behind the ears
• In the armpits
• In the groin
• At the backs of the hindlegs
• On the chin and neck
• Between the toes
• Along (especially under) the tail

GROOMING YOUR CAT

As soon as you obtain your cat, start a daily grooming routine. The range of equipment available is enormous so you may wish to ask the advice of a professional groomer, but the basic items that you will need are a brush, a comb and some moist face-wipes.

You will find grooming your cat easiest if he is relaxed: after a meal may be a good time. You may find it easiest to handle him if he is on a table. The amount of time that you should spend grooming your cat will depend on his coat, but ideally all cats should be groomed once a week, and given a quick 'tidy-up' as necessary.

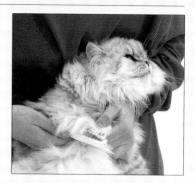

Grooming your cat will be easier if you use the correct techniques: ask a professional groomer for advice.

Short-haired cats are much less likely to develop fur mats than their longer-coated cousins.

Action

If you come across a mat of tangled hair when grooming your cat, do not try to 'snatch' a brush or comb through it. You will not clear the mat and you will hurt your cat. You should be able to tease apart a recently formed mat using your fingers or a metal comb.

For a more advanced mat, a tool called a mat-breaker is very useful. Holding the base of the mat with the fingers of one hand and the mat-breaker in the other, work at the mat from the edge and it will gradually come apart.

If your cat's coat is badly matted, seek the assistance of a professional cat-groomer: sometimes the only option is to shave off matted fur.

Prevention

Fur mats are an entirely preventable condition. Cats with different types of hair-coat need different amounts of coat care, but all cats will benefit from regular, thorough grooming.

A long-haired cat • First examine your cat's coat thoroughly. Look for any mats and tangles: there should not be any of these if you are grooming him regularly. Using a slicker brush (a pad of fine wire hooks) to remove loose hairs and debris trapped in his coat, and starting with your cat's legs, brush him gently but firmly, reaching down to the depths of his coat. Then move on to the sides of his body and between his legs, before tackling his back and tail. Finally, groom his head, neck and chest. Repeat the process using a comb to remove loose hairs. Finally, gently wipe away any discharge from around your cat's eyes and ear flaps using moist face-wipes.

A short-haired cat • Start with a bristle brush to remove dirt and to pull out any loose hairs. Then comb your cat's coat thoroughly, before cleaning his eyes and ear flaps using moist face-wipes.

Hypersensitivity reactions

These involve a complex chain of events that takes place as a cat's immune system over-reacts to the presence in or on his body of alien substances. Hypersensitivities are often referred to as allergies.

Cats may suffer from a number of hypersensitivity conditions that affect the skin; the most common of these are flea-bite hypersensitivity and atopy. Some cats may also have reactions to certain food items.

A cat may suffer from more than one type of hypersensitivity at the same time. In such a case, treatment that is given for only one kind of hypersensitivity may be sufficient to control the symptoms associated with the others.

FLEA-BITE HYPERSENSITIVITY

Fleas are very widespread, and a reaction to their feeding activities is the most common hypersensitivity condition (see also pages 54–6).

Causes

This condition is caused by an immune reaction in an affected cat to the saliva that a flea injects into his body while it is feeding.

Is it serious?

A severe hypersensitivity reaction can be very debilitating.

Cats at risk

This condition can affect cats of any age, breed or sex.

Action

If you notice any of the symptoms described, you should take your cat to be checked by your vet.

Your vet will examine your cat in detail. He or she will first look for evidence of fleas in his coat (see page 55), so do not groom your cat just before his appointment.

Your vet may then go on to carry out additional tests, as for atopy (see opposite).

Treatment

Treatment of an affected cat will normally be based on the following:
• The instigation of a rigorous flea-control campaign (see page 55).
• The use of anti-inflammatory medicines (see page 97).

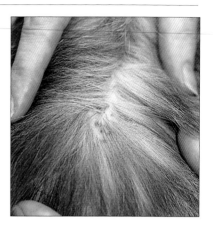

This cat is known to suffer from flea-bite hypersensitivity. The red spots on his skin are the first signs that he has been bitten again: without treatment, he will soon develop severe symptoms.

Even if flea control is rigorous and the cat does not suffer from any other hypersensitivities, symptoms may recur from time to time. Short-term use of anti-inflammatories may be prescribed as necessary, but long-term use should be avoided.

ATOPY

Atopy is an exaggerated response by a cat to certain substances in his environment, such as house dust, house-dust mites, and dandruff from humans and other animals. It results in marked skin irritation, and is the second most common hypersensitivity condition in cats.

Cats at risk

Atopy occurs in cats at any age, but symptoms often first appear from six months to two years of age.

Action

If you notice any of the symptoms described, take your cat to your vet as soon as possible.

COMMON SYMPTOMS

Flea-bite reactions in a hypersensitive cat are found most commonly on the lower back, hindlegs, inner thighs, abdomen, flanks and neck.
• Bite reactions typically form raised, crusty lumps that feel as though sugar has been sprinkled in the coat. This type of reaction is common to a number of other conditions, and is called miliary, or papulocrustous, dermatitis (see pages 58–9).
• Hypersensitivity reactions are intensely itchy, so an affected cat is likely to lick, nibble and scratch at his skin. As a result, he may develop further symptoms associated with self-trauma, such as alopecia as a result of excessive grooming (see pages 48–9) and obvious dandruff (skin scaling).
• Some cats may also develop eosinophilic granuloma complex lesions (see page 50).
• Affected cats tend to grow more hypersensitive as they age, so their symptoms may become more severe.

One in four cats with atopy may also be suffering from flea-bite and/or food hypersensitivity, so your vet will need to consider your cat's symptoms carefully. He or she will examine him meticulously, and will carry out a coat-brushing for evidence of fleas (see page 55).

To rule out the possibility of your cat's symptoms being due to flea-bite or food hypersensitivity, your vet may recommend that you first carry out a programme of rigorous flea control, and then feed him a special hypoallergenic diet for up to three months. If his symptoms do not improve in either case, this will suggest that your cat is suffering from atopy, so your vet may then carry out intradermal skin tests (see below) to identify any substances to which he may be hypersensitive.

Treatment

The symptoms of atopy can usually be controlled by appropriate treatment, including the following:
Avoidance • It will be very difficult to ensure that your cat is not exposed to the substances to which he is hypersensitive, but, depending on the results of the skin tests, your vet may suggest keeping your cat out of the house when you are cleaning, and that you do not allow him to sleep on carpets or stuffed furnishings.

COMMON SYMPTOMS

All cats suffering from atopy have itchy skin, and this generally continues all year round. The following are all common symptoms:
• Alopecia as a result of excessive self-grooming (see pages 48–9), without the underlying skin being inflamed. This is not always obvious to owners, as much of the grooming goes on in private. However, signs that the alopecia is self-inflicted may include evidence of vomited hair balls, tufts of hair in the cat's sleeping area, hair trapped between his teeth, or hair in his faeces.

• Eosinophilic granuloma complex lesions (see page 50).
• Miliary dermatitis (see pages 58–9)
• Symptoms associated with itchiness of the face, neck and ear flaps (such as excessive head-rubbing).
• As well as the cat's head and neck, other parts of the body that may show symptoms include the chest, abdomen, groin and thighs.
• Recurrent bouts of otitis externa (see pages 18–20).
• Bouts of sneezing
• Symptoms associated with skin infection (see pages 60–1).

Anti-inflammatory medicines • An effective treatment regime often involves the combined use of steroids (see page 97) or antihistamines, possibly with certain natural-oil preparations.
Shampoos and rinses • The use of special shampoos and rinses (your vet centre should supply these) may help to prevent dry skin and remove substances from the coat to which your cat is hypersensitive, but not all cats will tolerate bathing.
Anti-inflammatory cream • This may be given to relieve itchiness associated with small lesions, and so prevent symptoms from worsening through self-trauma.

Hyposensitization • This is a technique that aims to make the immune system less reactive to the substances that are causing the affected cat's condition.
Any treatment for a case of atopy will normally be required for life. One treatment regime may not be a permanent solution: your vet may need to adjust it from time to time.

FOOD HYPERSENSITIVITY

This is thought to be an immune reaction to specific proteins present in certain food items such as dairy products, fish, beef, pork, chicken, rabbit, lamb and eggs.

A cat who is affected will suffer from skin irritation, especially of his head, neck and ear flaps. Symptoms of this condition usually first appear at four to five years of age. Food hypersensitivity is less common than either flea-bite hypersensitivity or atopy.

Attempts at diagnosis, and a treatment regime, involve feeding a hypoallergenic diet for up to three months initially. Your vet will help you to plan a diet for your cat based on fresh ingredients or, better still, on prepared foods formulated for hypersensitive cats (see page 105).

INTRADERMAL SKIN TESTING

This is carried out to establish the substances to which a cat may be hypersensitive (it cannot be used to confirm food hypersensitivity). This type of test may only be undertaken after rigorous flea control and test-feeding with a hypoallergenic diet have been tried and assessed.

For the test, a cat will be sedated or anaesthetized (see pages 94–5), and an area of his skin will be clipped. Tiny amounts of substances known to be associated with hypersensitivities are then injected into the skin.

After a set time, the cat will be re-examined. An unusually large swelling found at any of the injection sites is considered a positive reaction, and suggests that the cat is hypersensitive to that particular substance.

Flea infestation

An infestation of fleas is a very common underlying cause of skin complaints in cats, in many parts of the world. These parasites are particularly prevalent during the spring and summer, although an abundance of centrally heated homes now means that they are an all-year-round pest in many places.

There are around 3000 different types of flea, including the dog flea, but the most common type found on cats – and dogs – is the cat flea.

Causes

Despite what many people think, fleas spend most of their lives in the environment, and not on cats. To these tiny creatures, cats and other warmblooded animals – such as dogs and people – are nothing more than roving restaurants.

An adult flea will jump on to a cat to feed, hanging on to his fur with its claws and biting through his skin to suck blood, using its needle-like mouthparts. A number of fleas are likely to have the same idea at the same time. While they are on the cat, they frantically mate and the females will lay hundreds of eggs. Within just a few days, the adult fleas die. The eggs drop to the ground, and in under two weeks a flea larva hatches from each one.

Over the next weeks to months the larva grows, feeding on mould, food crumbs, flakes of skin and even tapeworm eggs (see page 28). It then spins itself a cocoon shell, inside which it completely digests itself – brain, nervous system, guts and all – before building itself an adult body. As an adult, a flea can survive starvation for about eight months as it waits for a cat or dog meal to come along. The whole lifecycle may take up to two years.

THE LIFECYCLE OF THE FLEA

In one form or another, fleas spend most of their lives in the environment, only jumping on to a warmblooded animal – such as a cat – in order to feed and breed.

adult flea (on cat)

cocoon

eggs drop from cat's coat into environment

larva hatches from each egg

Your cat may pick up fleas from other cats, dogs and animals such as hedgehogs and rabbits, or from the environment in which these animals live, or which they visit. Fleas are able to breed extremely quickly: if your cat comes into your house one day with just 10 fleas on his back, within one month over 250,000 of them could have taken up residence with you.

Is it serious?

A flea infestation can be extremely debilitating for a cat, especially for a hypersensitive individual (see

---

COMMON SYMPTOMS

Fleas are visible to the naked eye, but it is fairly unusual to notice them in the environment unless an infestation is very bad. However, even if you cannot identify fleas on your cat, you may spot the telltale droppings that they will leave in his coat (see below).

Other symptoms of flea infestation include the following:
• Mild skin irritation as the fleas bite and scurry about: your cat may twitch his skin every now and again, or may groom and scratch himself more than normal. However, some cats show very little reaction to the attention of fleas.
• Severe skin irritation caused by an adverse reaction to flea saliva (see page 52). A hypersensitive cat is likely to feel extremely itchy and to indulge in excessive scratching, licking and fur-nibbling. He may end up with bald patches or areas of 'stubble hair' as a result, as well as tiny red lumps on his skin and dandruff (skin scaling).
• A severely affected cat may develop crusty spots, especially on his back, neck, base of his tail, inner thighs and abdomen. If your cat is hypersensitive to fleas, you will probably feel these spots before you see them.
• Symptoms that are associated with an intestinal tapeworm infestation (see page 28). Before it walls itself up in its cocoon, a flea larva may eat tapeworm eggs in the environment. A cat may swallow an adult flea when grooming and, as he digests it, the young tapeworm is freed to develop in his intestines.

page 52). Fleas are also the main source of tapeworm infestation in cats (see page 28).

Cats at risk

Any cat who has fleas in his environment is at risk of infestation.

Action

If your cat is showing any signs of skin irritation, check his coat for fleas and their telltale droppings. To do this, sit your cat on a sheet of white paper and then vigorously brush the fur on his back with your fingers. Specks of dirt and debris will fall on to the paper.

Moisten a cotton-wool pad with water, and dab it over the paper to pick up the debris. Wait for a few minutes, then look closely at the cotton wool. The blood contained in any flea droppings will dissolve and produce brown stains on the cotton wool.

If you find evidence of fleas on your cat, you should treat him, and more importantly your house, with appropriate insecticides, and then put into place a flea-prevention campaign (see page 56).

If you cannot find any evidence of fleas on your cat, take him to your vet. The symptoms that are associated with a flea infestation are very similar to those of other skin conditions, so your vet should examine your cat very thoroughly, and may repeat the coat-brushing procedure described above.

Treatment

If your vet finds evidence of a flea infestation on your cat, he or she is still likely to review your flea-prevention measures and to make any necessary adjustments. If

WARNING

Insecticides used to treat fleas are dangerous chemicals – they need to be, in order to work. Handle and use them with respect, and follow their instructions carefully.

You should never use more than one product at a time unless you are specifically instructed to do so by your vet.

Do not use products that are intended to control fleas in the environment on your cat.

your cats symptoms of irritation are severe, your vet may institute a rigorous flea-control programme, even if he or she cannot find evidence of fleas.

If this does not help, your vet may then go on to carry out a test feed trial and intradermal skin tests if necessary (see page 53).

If at all possible, your vet will avoid the use of anti-inflammatory medicines – such as steroids – (see

If you have a look through your cat's coat and cannot see any fleas, do not assume that they are not there: adult fleas can be difficult to spot. Instead, you should sit your cat on a sheet of white paper and carry out a coat-brushing (left). When dabbed up on to a dampened cotton-wool pad, flea droppings will dissolve to produce obvious brown stains of dried blood (below).

page 97). Although they will stop your cat scratching, they will make it impossible for your vet to assess whether flea control is beneficial to his condition.

Prevention

Implementing a flea-prevention campaign should be a routine part of caring for your cat. You should do the following:

• Regularly vacuum-clean and then wash all your cat's bedding.

• Regularly vacuum-clean your house (placing an insecticidal collar inside the bag may help to kill any adult fleas that hatch out inside it).

• Spray around your house with an insecticide designed to kill adult fleas. The best products also stop flea eggs from developing into adults and only need to be used a few times a year.

• Regularly treat your cat, together with any other cats or dogs who live with him, with insecticidal products made for them.

There are many flea-treatment products from which to choose, including sprays, powders, foams, shampoos, skin drops, preparations to give by mouth (see pages 101–2) and insecticidal collars.

The ways in which these flea products work differ, and no single product is perfect for all cats (for instance, some are unsuitable for use on young kittens or on pregnant cats). You should ask at your vet centre for advice about the most suitable products to use in your house and on your cat, and when you should use them.

Sprays, powders and shampoos • These kill fleas that come into contact with a cat's coat.

Skin drops and oral medication • Liquids given as a few drops on the skin and medications given by mouth are absorbed into the blood, and a flea has to suck this to be killed by the insecticide. For cats who are allergic to flea saliva, the fleas must be killed

before they bite, so these methods may be unsuitable.

Insecticidal collars • If you use one of these on your cat, make sure that it is designed to expand or break should a stick or other object become caught under it while your cat is out and about.

Ultrasonic devices • These are designed to repel fleas, and their makers claim that they are silent to cats. However, research has shown that cats can hear them, so do not use such a device on your cat or in your home.

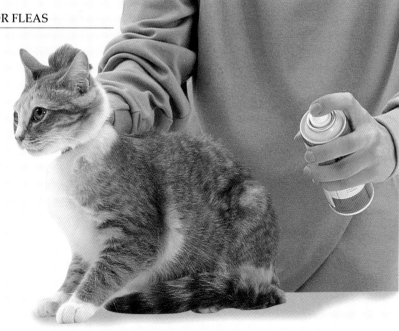

SPRAYING A CAT FOR FLEAS

Sprays can be difficult to use because many cats hate the sound that they make. The easiest and safest way to hold your cat for spraying is to place him on a table and then to grasp him by his scruff (see pages 99–100). Fluff up your cat's coat with your free hand before spraying him.

If your cat tries to scratch you with a hindleg, lift his front end off the table by his scruff. With some cats, it may be necessary to lift them completely off the table for a few seconds while spraying them. If you do this, your cat may curl up his feet, as young kittens do when they are carried in their mothers' mouths.

Despite what many owners think, cats are relatively easy to spray if the correct technique is used.

Other skin parasites

A cat's skin and coat may become home to a number of parasites in addition to fleas. The creatures that may be parasitic on your cat will depend on the area or country in which you live, but the following are some of the most common skin parasites of cats.

LICE

An infestation of a cat with lice is called pediculosis. Lice are small, flattened, wingless insects, and are spread from cat to cat through close contact or on shared grooming tools and bedding. They can only survive for a few days away from a cat.

Lice can be seen by the naked eye, but using a magnifying glass makes it easier to identify both the lice themselves and their eggs (called nits), which remain firmly attached to individual hairs. Lice are easily killed through routine insecticidal treatments used to control fleas (see opposite).

Cats most likely to suffer from pediculosis are those living in unhygienic conditions, those with ungroomed and matted coats (see page 51), individuals who are old or sick, and cats who live together in overcrowded conditions.

Some cats may carry lice without showing any adverse symptoms,

This is a highly magnified picture of a cat louse. It uses its biting mouthparts to feed on a cat's skin debris and hair.

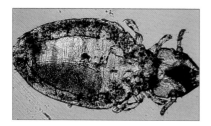

but others may show the following signs of an infestation:
• A 'mousey' smell to the coat
• Signs of miliary dermatitis (see pages 58–9)
• A cat who is very itchy is likely to show symptoms associated with self-trauma (see pages 48–9).

TICKS

Ticks are eight-legged creatures that are related to spiders. The ticks most commonly found on cats are 'castor-bean' or 'sheep' ticks, and also 'hedgehog' ticks. They have leathery bodies and spend most of their lives in the environment, only visiting cats or other animals to feed for periods of a few days during the spring or autumn. Ticks may live for up to three years, and a female may lay a staggering 8000 eggs in her lifetime.

Cats pick up ticks by brushing against tick-infested plants. Ticks are visible to the naked eye, but their bodies are often mistaken for small warts or cysts when their heads are buried in a cat's skin. Their bodies become most obvious when they enlarge after feeding.

Through their feeding activities, certain ticks may spread serious infections, and may also provoke the following symptoms:
• Skin irritation
• Anaemia (in a heavy infestation)

MITES

Mites are tiny creatures and, like ticks, are also related to spiders. The following are all mites that affect cats in the UK.

Cheyletiella mites

These mites spend their whole lives on the outer surface of an affected cat's skin. A cat normally becomes

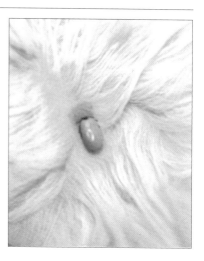

A tick in a cat's skin will be visible to the naked eye, especially when its body has enlarged after a meal of blood.

infested through direct contact with an infested cat or other animal, and may suffer from severe dandruff (skin scaling) and/or symptoms of miliary dermatitis (see pages 58–9).

Ear mites
(See page 20.)

Harvest mites

These are common in grassland, especially on chalky ground. Only the bright orange, young mites are parasitic to cats, dogs and other animals when they emerge in late summer and autumn. Cats pick up harvest mites from the ground, and their presence on their feet, legs, heads and ears may cause severe irritation and symptoms of miliary dermatitis (see pages 58–9).

FLIES

The adult forms of many flies may lay their eggs on the warm, wet skin of cats who are debilitated, who are suffering from skin wounds or who have urine-soaked coats. The larvae that develop from the eggs can cause severe skin inflammation and tissue damage. An infestation with fly larvae is known as myiasis or 'fly strike'.

Action

To remove a tick from your cat's skin, first dab the tick with a piece of cotton wool wetted with an appropriate insecticide; some flea sprays (see page 56) also kill ticks . Leave the tick for a few minutes to die, then grasp it near the skin with a pair of tweezers, rotate it through a quarter-turn and 'unplug' it by pulling gently. Do not snatch at the tick, or you may leave its biting mouthparts embedded in your cat's skin, resulting in inflammation and possible infection.

Take your cat to your vet if you are unable to remove a tick, or if you have spotted any parasites (other than fleas) but do not know what they are. Do not use flea treatments on your cat beforehand (see page 56), as these may kill other parasites, making diagnosis difficult for your vet.

To confirm the identity of any skin parasite, your vet will examine your cat very thoroughly. He or she may then carry out specific tests, such as taking hair and dandruff samples for detailed examination under a microscope.

Treatment

All cats with a parasite infestation require prompt and thorough treatment. In most cases this will involve the use of chemicals to kill the parasites. Your vet may also prescribe medicines to control symptoms such as inflammation: this may be associated directly with the infestation, or may have occurred as a result of self-trauma through your cat's attempts to relieve the irritation that he feels.

Ticks or fly larvae on your cat must be removed individually.

ZOONOSIS

Many of the skin parasites that affect cats – such as cheyletiella and harvest mites – will also cause occasional symptoms in people. If you or members of your family have any unusual bite marks on your body that you are not able to explain, contact your doctor. You should also arrange for your cat to be checked by your vet, even if he is not showing obvious symptoms.

Prevention

If you live in an area known to be tick-infested (your vet centre will be able to advise you), you should incorporate measures to control ticks into your flea-prevention campaign (see page 56). Grooming your cat regularly will enable you to spot signs of skin parasites as soon as they appear, so that you can treat your cat and prevent him from suffering unnecessarily.

Miliary dermatitis

Miliary dermatitis – also known as papulocrustous dermatitis – is a term that is used to describe the appearance on a cat's skin of multiple crusty lesions.

Causes

This inflammatory reaction of the skin is common to a range of underlying conditions including:
• Flea infestation (see pages 54–6)
• Lice infestation (see pages 57–8)
• Mite infestations, such as ear mites (see page 20) and cheyletiella or harvest mites (see pages 57–8).
• Hypersensitivity skin conditions, including flea-bite hypersensitivity, atopy and food hypersensitivity (see pages 52–3).
• Dermatophytosis (see page 49)

As many as eight out of 10 cases of miliary dermatitis in cats are thought to be the result of flea-bite hypersensitivity, but in some cases no underlying cause is identified.

Is it serious?

Miliary dermatitis is an irritating and uncomfortable condition for a cat. In addition, the longer a case is left untreated, the more severe the symptoms will become and the more difficult it may be for your vet to identify the underlying cause. For this reason, all cases should be taken seriously.

Cats at risk

All cats are at risk of suffering from miliary dermatitis.

Action

If your cat exhibits any of the symptoms described, you should arrange for him to be examined by your vet as soon as possible.

Your vet's aim will be to identify the underlying cause of the miliary dermatitis, in order to be able to prescribe appropriate and specific treatment. The investigations that may be needed will take time, so be patient and do not expect a miracle cure at your cat's first appointment.

Your vet be able to prescribe medicines that will alleviate the symptoms of this condition in just a few days, but the symptoms will quickly recur if the underlying cause has not been resolved.

The fur over this miliary dermatitis lesion has been shaved, making it easy to see that the skin is crusty and scabby, and covered in many small bumps.

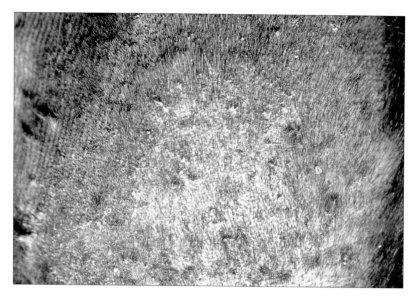

There may be several stages to the investigation of your cat's symptoms, which may involve:
• Physical examination
• Analysis of coat brushings, and of skin and hair samples, to look for dermatophytosis (see page 49), evidence of fleas (see pages 54–6) and other common skin parasites (see pages 57–8).
• Evaluation of his response to aggressive flea control, both on him and in your house (see page 56).
• Evaluation of your cat's response to a hypoallergenic diet for a period of up to three months (see page 53).
• Intradermal skin tests to check for allergies (see page 53).

Treatment

If your vet is able to identify the underlying cause of the miliary dermatitis, he or she will institute a specific treatment (and, if necessary, a prevention) regime.

Once the cause has been brought under control, the crusty lesions and other symptoms shown should quickly start to resolve.

To help speed up recovery if a specific cause has been confirmed, or if the cause remains unidentified despite tests, your vet may resort to a short course of powerful anti-inflammatory medicines, such as steroids (see page 97).

If a cause cannot be identified, repeated courses of medication may be needed as and when symptoms recur, or even on a permanent basis (at the lowest dose rate possible) if your cat begins to suffer again as soon as the treatment is stopped.

Aftercare

During the period that your cat's symptoms are being investigated, he will still feel uncomfortable and possibly irritable. Anxiety, boredom and over-warm conditions appear to make the itchiness worse in many cases, so you should try to ensure that your cat's life is stress-free but interesting, and give him the option of sleeping in a cooler environment than normal if he wishes. You should also try to avoid handling and fussing him unless he is the one to initiate the attention.

You must strictly follow any instructions from your vet about your cat's dietary regime and any flea-prevention measures that you should undertake on your cat and in your house (see also page 56).

Prevention

As flea-bite hypersensitivity is the underlying cause most frequently identified in cases of miliary dermatitis, you should adopt a thorough and well-planned flea-prevention campaign from the time that you first bring your cat home to live with you.

COMMON SYMPTOMS

The crusty lesions may appear in just one small area, or over a large extent of a cat's body in a severe case. The lesions can be felt as tiny lumps in the skin, and the crusts that are produced in association with them may feel as though sugar has been sprinkled in the coat. Other symptoms may include the following:
• Skin twitching, due to irritation
• Areas of alopecia (see pages 48–9), due to the cat's excessive grooming and scratching attempts to relieve irritation; such areas may contain broken, 'stubble' hairs.
• Other symptoms associated with excessive grooming and nibbling, including vomited hair balls, fur trapped between the teeth, and fur appearing in the cat's faeces.
• Obvious temperament changes, such as general restlessness and/or aggression when handled.
• Some cats also exhibit symptoms of eosinophilic granuloma complex (see page 50) at the same time.

Subcutaneous abscess

A subcutaneous abscess is a pocket of pus that accumulates under a cat's skin, as a result of a bacterial infection. This condition is one of the most common reasons for cats being taken to their vet centres for medical attention.

Causes

Most subcutaneous abscesses occur in cats as a result of penetrating bite wounds sustained during fights.

When one cat bites another, bacteria that are normally present in the mouth are injected by the canine teeth as they penetrate the victim's skin. There may be one or more bite holes, which are usually very small and quickly seal up: the only evidence may be a tiny tuft of hairs stuck together by a scab where each bite hole was made.

A localized infection may then develop over the next two to four

Subcutaneous abscesses in cats are often referred to simply as cat-bite abscesses, as most occur as a result of fights.

COMMON SYMPTOMS

• An abscess may appear as a soft swelling or may rupture, discharging copious quantities of foul-smelling yellow-green pus.
• Most abscesses are painful, and a cat may well resent handling of the area.
• Sometimes the infection resulting from a cat bite remains deepseated and spreads through the tissue in the area, rather than forming a discrete abscess. This type of skin infection, or pyoderma, is called cellulitis, and results in skin that is usually swollen, discoloured and foul-smelling.
• A cat with an abscess on one of his legs may be lame (see page 47).

days. This may be contained and controlled by the cat's immune system, but will often turn into an abscess under the skin. Most cat-bite abscesses occur around the base of the tail, on the neck and around the shoulders.

Is it serious?

Most abscesses will resolve with aggressive treatment. However, an abscess under the skin may be a cause of other serious infections such as exudative pleurisy (see page 37), so prompt treatment for all skin abscesses is essential.

Bite wounds are also a common means by which two of the major infectious diseases to affect cats – feline immunodeficiency virus infection and feline leukaemia virus infection (see pages 80–3) – may be transmitted from an infected cat to a healthy one.

Cats at risk

All cats are at risk of suffering from subcutaneous abscesses, but bite wounds sustained from fighting with other cats are most commonly found in adult male cats who are able to roam freely outdoors.

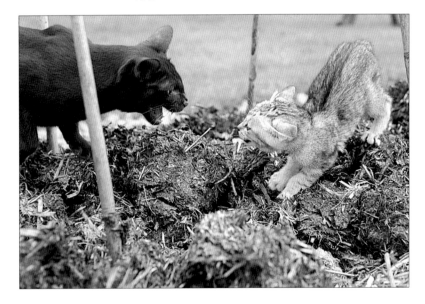

ZOONOSIS

If any cat bites or scratches you and you subsequently develop a small skin lesion rather like an insect-bite reaction, you should contact your doctor.

So called cat-scratch disease is now a well-recognized condition in people, and affected individuals can become very ill, normally about three weeks after having been scratched or bitten.

The organism responsible for this disease remains unknown. The cat who has done the biting may not even be the source of the organism involved, but may simply pass it on.

Action

If you think or know that your cat has been involved in a fight with another cat, examine him closely to look for bite wounds. You should ask someone else to help you to restrain your cat properly while you do this (see pages 98–100).

The easiest way to locate a bite wound is to feel through your cat's coat with the tips of your fingers. If you reach a spot that he resents you handling, check that area closely for blood-stained hairs, then part the fur and look for the tiny bite-wound holes. If you find any wounds, cut off a little fur over them – using curved scissors – so that you can identify their position again.

Bathe any bite wounds with warm, salty water and then with a veterinary antiseptic solution. Pick off any scabs that form, to keep the wounds open: if they seal too quickly, an abscess may be more likely to appear. Keep your cat indoors, and bathe his wounds frequently over the next few days. He may recover without further incident, but, if a swelling begins to develop, the wound area remains painful or your cat is unwell in any other way, take him to your vet as soon as possible.

If the fight occurred several days earlier, your cat may have an obvious swelling, or may be lame (see page 47). Any wounds will have sealed up by this stage, so feel instead for small tufts of hair stuck together. If you locate a tuft, pull it out in one swift movement.

Beneath it will be a bite-wound hole, and, if an abscess has already started to form, your efforts may well be rewarded with a flow of foul-smelling pus. In this case, clean up any discharge and bathe the wound carefully (see above), before contacting your vet centre.

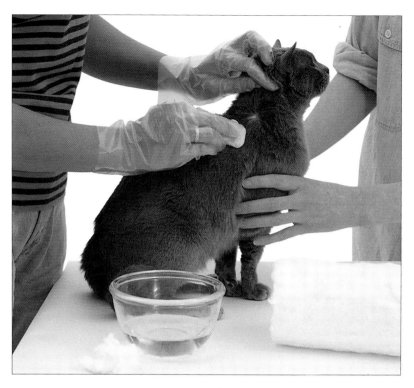

If your cat has a bite (or claw) wound, ask someone to restrain him. Bathe the area with warm, salty water, followed by a veterinary antiseptic solution.

If you have not identified any wound holes, your vet will look for them. He or she will also examine your cat thoroughly in order to check for any other symptoms that you may have missed.

Treatment

If the infection is mild and has not developed into a full-blown abscess, your vet may simply treat your cat with antibiotics: a course lasting from five to seven days is normally sufficient.

If your cat has an advanced abscess, your vet may admit him to the vet centre for an anaesthetic (see pages 94–5), so that he can lance the abscess and then flush it out with antibiotic solutions.

Aftercare

At home, you will need to keep your cat indoors until he has fully recovered, to administer prescribed antibiotics (see pages 101–2), and to bathe any bite or surgical wounds according to your vet's instructions.

Prevention

If cat fights are common in your area, keep your cat indoors at dawn and dusk (the times at which the most dominant male cats in the neighbourhood will be patrolling their territories) to reduce your cat's chances of being involved in a fight.

In my view, all male (tom) cats who are not destined for breeding should be castrated, at the age of about six months. This will not only reduce the number of unwanted pregnancies in female cats, but will also reduce the desire of the males to roam and to fight other cats who cross their paths.

Solar dermatitis

Solar dermatitis is a chronic, or long-term, inflammatory condition of white-haired areas of skin, most commonly on the face and ear flaps. The disease generally occurs in cats living in warm climates, and may begin when an individual is just three months old. However, it can also appear in older cats who live in more temperate regions.

Causes

The cause of solar dermatitis is the repeated exposure to ultraviolet (UVB) light from the sun's rays.

Is it serious?

If it is left untreated, the affected skin may become cancerous (see pages 68–9). This usually occurs when an affected cat is over six years old, but may happen earlier in some cases. This type of cancer,

If you live in a sunny climate and your cat has white ears, cover their tips with sunblock before he goes outdoors.

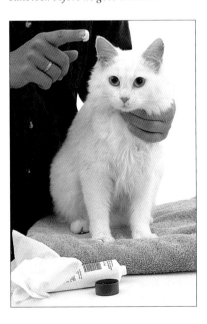

which is called squamous-cell carcinoma, causes ulceration and bleeding and may destroy the edges of affected ear flaps.

Cats at risk

Solar dermatitis is most common in white cats, or on the white-haired areas of cats who have coloured coats. White cats who have blue eyes seem particularly susceptible to this condition.

Action

If your cat exhibits any of the symptoms described, you should arrange for him to be examined by your vet as soon as possible. He or she will start by examining your cat thoroughly. To confirm that he is suffering from solar dermatitis, and to rule out other causes of similar symptoms, your vet may need to take a biopsy of affected skin (see page 92) for laboratory analysis.

Treatment

If your cat is diagnosed as having solar dermatitis, his treatment regime may involve the following:

Avoidance of sunlight • You should not allow your cat to go outdoors during the main hours of sunlight, or to sunbathe near open windows or doors.

Sunscreens • During the summer months, you should cover the vulnerable areas of your cat's skin with waterproof sunblock.

Medication • Your vet may prescribe medicines containing substances called carotenoids: these are thought to help make compounds in the skin that can absorb damaging radiation.

Surgery • Your vet may need to operate on your cat in order to remove part or all of an affected

COMMON SYMPTOMS

• Reddening of an affected area of skin
• Very fine scaling of the skin at the edges of an affected ear flap
• Lesions will gradually become more severe over subsequent summers: the skin will become redder and more inflamed, the scaling will worsen and crusts will form. An affected cat may cause further damage by scratching the lesions to relieve the discomfort and pain that he feels. At this stage, the margins of the eyelids, nose and lips may also be affected.

ear flap, if the results of biopsy analysis (see page 92) reveal that irreversible changes have occurred in the skin. This may simply involve removing the very edge of the ear flap, but in a severe case amputation of the entire ear flap may be necessary. By controlling your cat's exposure to the sun, using sunblock creams and administering any prescribed medication (see pages 101–2), you will play a crucial part in helping to treat and manage his condition.

Prevention

If you have a cat with white-haired ears and you live in a sunny region, cover his ears with sunblock before he goes out in the sun. You should ask for your vet's advice, or contact the manufacturer of any cream that you intend to use, to ensure that your cat will not come to any harm if he should ingest small amounts of it when he grooms himself.

Ideally, you should encourage a white-haired cat to stay indoors in the daytime during the sunniest periods of the year.

Claw conditions

Claws, or nails, are dead, horny structures on the ends of each of the toes. Normal cats have five toes on each front paw, and four on each back paw. The front claws are covered by sheaths of skin, but the cat can expose them at will.

Of the many claw disorders to affect cats, overlong and broken or torn claws are the most common.

Causes

Overlong claws are caused by insufficient wear. A cat's claws grow all the time, but under normal circumstances they are constantly worn down through wear and tear. Although the claws on the front toes are covered by skin much of the time, a normal, active cat who claws at objects outside, or who uses a scratching-post indoors, will keep his claws at the correct length and honed to sharp points. He should also keep the claws on his hind paws in perfect condition through his normal activity.

As a result, overlong claws are usually only a problem in cats who do not engage in normal activity (for example, as a result of illness or old age, or because they live indoors and are not provided with a scratching-post). They may also occur in cats with abnormal claw growth, such as those who have hyperthyroidism (see page 72).

Physical damage to the claws is common, and will be more likely to occur if the claws are overlong.

Is it serious ?

Overlong nails may affect the way a cat walks and his ability to climb, and may make him more prone to injuries such as joint sprains. If left untreated, overlong claws will eventually grow around and bury

A CAT'S CLAW

Each of a cat's claws should be honed to a sharp point. In clipping an overlong claw, care must be taken not to cut into the sensitive quick; sharp 'guillotine'-type clippers should be used.

normal claw   overlong claw

themselves deep into the toe pads, causing infection and severe pain.

Infection of the soft tissues that surround each claw occurs most commonly following claw damage.

Action

Overlong claws • If you think that your cat's claws may be too long, ask your vet, a veterinary nurse or a professional cat-groomer to look at them. If the claws are too long, he or she will very carefully clip them for you. If because of your cat's lifestyle or rapid claw growth the problem may recur, ask for a demonstration of how to clip his claws properly and safely yourself.

A broken claw • If the snapped tip of a claw is hanging off, but the claw is not bleeding and does not

COMMON SYMPTOMS

Overlong and broken claws are obvious; other symptoms may include the following:
• Lameness (see page 47) due to pain, especially with a broken claw
• Resentment of a paw or paws being handled in any way

look raw, you may be able to clip it free. As the toe may be painful, you must have an assistant to restrain your cat properly (see pages 98–100). If the claw is very badly damaged – especially if it is bleeding – bandage the paw (see page 109), then take your cat to your vet as soon as possible.

Treatment

If your cat has a seriously damaged claw, your vet may need to remove the broken part or even the entire claw. If there is bacterial infection of the tissues around the claw, your vet will prescribe antibiotics.

Aftercare

After surgery you must keep your cat indoors for several days. You may be asked by your vet to change his dressings (see page 109).

Prevention

Check the length of your cat's claws as part of routine health-checks (see pages 8–9), and give him the chance to wear them down through natural clawing activity: if he is an indoor cat, you must provide at least one scratching-post. You may need to trim his hind claws occasionally.

Kidneys and bladder

A cat's urinary system consists of the two kidneys and bladder, the ureters (small tubes) that connect them, and the urethra through which urine is emptied from the bladder. There are two serious conditions that commonly affect the urinary system of cats. In a case of renal failure, the two kidneys – despite the in-built spare working capacity that they have – are so affected by disease that they cannot carry out their normal functions, while feline lower-urinary-tract disease involves a cat's bladder and urethra.

Renal failure

A cat's two kidneys have several vital functions, including removal of the waste products of protein-processing from the body, and a role in maintaining the body's water levels and of the chemical substances dissolved in that water.

The filter-like working parts of a kidney are called nephrons, each of which consists of a blood filter attached to a complex piece of pipework called a tubule.

Both of the kidneys contain hundreds of thousands of neprons. When a significant number of them become damaged or are destroyed by disease, such that the remaining nephrons cannot cope, the cat will suffer from renal failure.

Causes

In many cases, the underlying disease that is responsible for renal failure remains unknown, but the following are all possible causes:
• Development problems affecting the kidneys, called congenital renal conditions, that are present at birth (these are uncommon).
• Chronic interstitial nephritis, or inflammation of the internal structure of the kidneys. This is a progressive disease, thought to be one of the more common causes of renal failure in older cats. Its cause is not fully understood.
• Bacterial infection of the kidneys.
• An inflammation of the blood-filtering parts of kidney nephrons

called glomerulonephritis, which is the result of certain complex immune-system processes.
• Cancer of the kidneys, especially lymphomas (see pages 68–9).
• Amyloidosis: this affects kidney tubules, and may occur due to long-term immune-system reactions to diseases of other body parts.
• Feline infectious peritonitis (see page 82).
• Damage to the kidneys as a result of poisoning: for instance, by some types of anti-freeze (see page 120).
• Obstruction to the normal flow of urine – for example, by uroliths in a male cat (see pages 66–7) – causing a pressure build-up in the kidneys that is damaging to the nephrons.
• Direct damage to the kidneys, as a result of severe trauma.

• The kidneys take about 25 per cent of the blood pumped from a cat's heart, and renal failure may occur due to any disorder – such as severe dehydration – that reduces the blood supply to the kidneys.

Renal failure may be termed acute or chronic. In acute renal failure, a significant number of nephrons all stop working at the same time, as may occur in sudden urinary blockages. Chronic renal failure occurs more gradually due to progressive underlying diseases, and is the most common type of renal failure to affect cats.

Is it serious?

Renal failure is a life-threatening condition. The long-term outlook for most cats with chronic renal

COMMON SYMPTOMS

Even though the disease that incites chronic renal failure may have been present for many years, symptoms often seem to appear suddenly.

The reason for this is that a cat can survive without showing any symptoms of kidney problems even when the whole of one kidney and one-third of the other have been put out of action. In chronic renal failure, the damage to the kidneys is usually irreversible and progressive.

The symptoms of renal failure may include the following:

• Weight loss
• Reluctance to eat
• Increased urine production
• Altered drinking habits: increased thirst (resulting from increased urine production) may drive your cat to drink in unusual places, such as from a pond or even from the toilet.
• Gingivitis (see pages 24–5)
• Vomiting (see pages 26–7)
• Pale gums (see page 75)
• Bad breath
• Poor coat condition
• Depression and lethargy

THE ANATOMY OF A CAT'S KIDNEY

A cat's kidneys are bean-shaped organs, about half the size of the one shown here. Blood enters through the renal artery, is filtered within the kidney tissue and leaves through the renal vein. The urine produced by this process passes through the nephrons, then from the kidney to the bladder through the ureter.

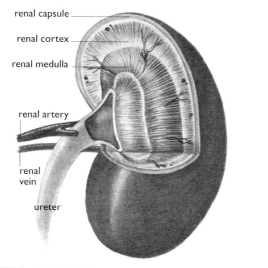

renal capsule

renal cortex

renal medulla

renal artery

renal vein

ureter

failure is poor, but many can enjoy a good quality of life if treatment is initiated promptly, and is diligently carried out by the cats' owners.

Cats at risk

All cats are at risk. However, the symptoms of renal failure are most commonly seen in older cats, in whom the diseases responsible for the condition may have been established for years (see opposite).

Action

If your cat exhibits any of the symptoms described, take him to your vet as soon as possible.

Your vet will consider the history of your cat's symptoms and will examine him thoroughly. He or she is likely to pay particular attention to feeling the size and shape of his kidneys through palpating his abdomen as, with renal failure, the kidneys may be enlarged, or small and shrunken.

Your vet will also carry out blood tests (in particular to look for raised levels of urea, a waste product of

protein-processing within the body), and may also carry out urine tests, X-ray and ultrasound investigations. In exceptional cases, a biopsy of a kidney may be taken for examination (see pages 91–2).

Treatment

In most cases of renal failure the cause is not identified, so your vet may only be able to begin treatment aimed at alleviating the symptoms.

Intensive care • If your cat is very ill, your vet will admit him as an in-patient until he is fit enough to be nursed at home. If your cat has stopped drinking and

WARNING

If your cat is known to suffer from renal failure but suddenly shows new symptoms, contact your vet immediately. Other conditions, which would be deemed trivial in a healthy cat, could seriously affect his renal problems and will require prompt and aggressive treatment.

is dehydrated, he will need fluids via a 'drip' (see page 93).

Dietary management • A cat who has renal failure may benefit from alterations in the protein, fat, mineral and vitamin levels in his diet. Your vet or a veterinary nurse will put together a feeding plan (including times of meals), which is likely to include prepared foods formulated for use in the management of renal failure (see page 105). If your cat's appetite is depressed, you may need to encourage him to eat (see pages 104–5).

Medication • The use of specific medicines may help to resolve any associated problems such as vomiting (see pages 26–7), anaemia (see page 75) and lack of appetite.

Chemotherapy • This is an option for cats who are suffering from lymphoma (see pages 68–9).

A cat with chronic renal failure will require treatment for life. Initially, when symptoms are mild, this may simply involve changes to his diet. As the underlying cause of his renal failure progresses, his treatment is likely to become more involved, and your vet will want to monitor his condition on a regular basis (this may involve repeated blood or other tests).

Aftercare

At home, you must ensure that your cat has permanent access to fresh water. Your vet may suggest adding water to your cat's food or offering him broth or even milk if he is able to digest it, to encourage his voluntary fluid intake.

You must also help your cat to lead a stress-free life, by trying to prevent him over-exerting himself and keeping him warm (but not hot). It may be appropriate for you to keep him indoors.

Feline lower-urinary-tract disease

This is more of a syndrome than a single condition. It affects the lower urinary tract, which consists of the bladder and urethra (the tube that carries urine from the bladder), and is often simply called FLUTD.

No matter what the underlying cause, the symptoms are often very similar. They are usually associated with inflammation of the inner lining of the bladder (or cystitis), and with partial or complete blockage of the urethra (almost always in male cats).

Causes

The underlying conditions involved in lower-urinary-tract disease are still not fully understood, and this syndrome of the cat is the subject of ongoing study.

However, in as many as one in five cats suffering from FLUTD, the underlying problem is thought to be a condition called urolithiasis. This involves the formation within the urinary system of microscopic mineral crystals that develop into deposits called uroliths, either in the form of a sand-like substance, or as discrete 'stones'.

The most common type of urolith consists of magnesium ammonium phosphate, more commonly referred to as struvite. The reasons why struvite forms in the first place are complex, but its appearance in a cat's bladder is thought to be influenced by his diet, his feeding regime and his body's processing of water. It seems that the effect of a cat's overall dietary regime on the acidity of his urine is of particular importance.

As well as uroliths, so-called 'urethral plugs' may form in a cat's lower urinary tract. These also contain mineral crystals – most commonly struvite – mixed with other materials such as blood cells, sperm and/or organisms such as viruses and bacteria.

The second most common type of uroliths found in cats are made of a substance called calcium oxalate. The reasons for the formation of these has been less well-studied.

Bacterial infections may help to complicate feline lower-urinary-tract disease, but such infections are rarely the initial cause.

Is it serious?

Even at its mildest, feline lower-urinary-tract disease must be assumed to be an uncomfortable and possibly a painful condition.

Without prompt treatment, it may also lead on to more serious complications. For instance, some cats – especially male cats – may go on to develop complete urinary blockages due to urolithiasis, and may suffer from renal failure (see pages 64–5) within 24 to 48 hours as a result, if left untreated.

Cats at risk

Although they are not proven, a number of factors may predispose a cat to suffer from feline lower-urinary-tract disease, including inactivity (in many cases, this is associated with confinement indoors), obesity (see pages 76–7), castration or spaying, a diet of dry food and a low fluid intake.

For unknown reasons, long-haired cats may be more prone to this condition, while Siamese cats may be less at risk of it than other breeds. Male cats, with their much narrower urethras, are more likely to suffer from urinary obstruction.

Action

If your cat shows any abnormalities relating either to how or where he urinates, or to what he produces, keep him indoors and take him to your vet as soon as possible. If he keeps straining to pass urine but does not produce anything, contact your vet centre as an emergency.

Your vet will examine your cat, and will wish to carry out urine tests (see page 92). For these, he or she may take a sample from your cat's bladder through his body wall, using a syringe and needle, or may provide you with a special litter-tray to collect a sample at home. Your vet may also carry out blood tests (especially if your cat has a urinary obstruction), and may take X-ray pictures of his abdomen.

COMMON SYMPTOMS

Precise symptoms vary, but many are due to inflammation of the bladder wall (cystitis), or to the presence of complete or partial obstructions to normal urine flow. They may include the following:
• More frequent urination than is normal.
• Apparent difficulty and discomfort in passing small amounts of urine.

• Blood-tinged urine
• Urination in unusual places, such as 'accidents' indoors.
• Straining without the production of any urine (almost always in male cats). A cat who shows this symptom may be suffering from a complete urinary obstruction that may quickly lead to symptoms associated with renal failure (see pages 64–5).

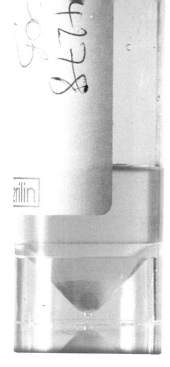

This is a urine sample from a healthy cat. It has been allowed to stand, but has remained clear. If your vet asks you to collect a urine sample from your cat at home, he or she should provide you with a special false-bottomed litter-tray.

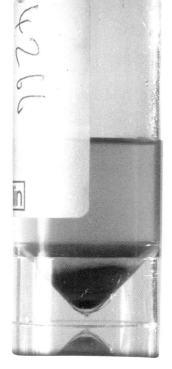

This urine sample has been taken from a cat with urolithiasis. It has been left to stand, and blood has started to settle at the bottom of the container. This blood in the urine is due to inflammation of the bladder lining, or cystitis.

Treatment

If tests reveal an obstruction of your cat's urinary system, your vet will carry out emergency procedures before starting investigations into a possible underlying cause. This will mean anaesthetizing your cat (see pages 94–5) before trying to unblock the urethra.

If the blockage is at the tip of the penis of a male cat, it may be fairly easy to remove. However, if it is further towards his bladder, your vet will try to clear it by passing a tiny tube, called a urinary catheter, up his urethra and then flushing special fluid through it. If this proves to be unsuccessful, your vet may have to operate.

If your cat is not suffering from a urinary obstruction when your vet examines him, or a blockage within his urinary system has been successfully cleared by surgery,

your vet will initiate a treatment regime that is aimed at resolving any underlying cause.

Resolving urolithiasis • In the case of urolithiasis or urethral-plug formation due to struvite 'sand' or 'stones', the treatment may involve administering special medicines to make the cat's urine more acidic, and adding extra water to his diet to increase his fluid intake and promote a greater urine flow.

Dietary adaptation • Alternatively (and preferably), your vet may recommend changing your cat on to a diet formulated to help treat lower-urinary-tract disease (see page 105). This will not only help to increase the amount of urine produced and make it more acidic, but will also provide levels of both magnesium and phosphorus in line with current

recommendations to prevent the formation of struvite. On such a diet, symptoms may resolve within a matter of days as any struvite – even in the form of discrete uroliths in the bladder – begins to dissolve. However, if your cat is suffering from urolithiasis as a result of other kinds of urolith (for example, those made of calcium oxalate), your vet may wish to operate to remove any uroliths that may be present in your cat's bladder.

Antibiotics • Your vet will prescribe these if he or she believes that bacterial infection may be involved.

Despite investigation, the cause of FLUTD may remain unknown. Treatment in such cases is likely to involve dietary modifications.

Aftercare

If your cat has had an anaesthetic and/or surgery, your vet or a veterinary nurse should give you specific instructions about his nursing care at home (see also pages 98–111). You must be sure to follow your vet's specific dietary recommendations very carefully, and to take your cat back to your vet centre for check-ups and repeat tests as necessary.

Prevention

Urolithiasis as a result of struvite formation may recur in as many as seven out of 10 cats. If your cat does suffer from this condition, it is therefore likely that your vet will recommend making long-term changes to his diet to help prevent the formation of new uroliths.

You can help by encouraging your cat to lead an active life and to drink plenty of water. As obesity can be a factor, you must also aim to keep your cat at his ideal weight (see pages 76–7).

Other important conditions

Various types of cancer, diabetes mellitus (often referred to as 'sugar diabetes'), hyperthyroidism, rupture of the diaphragm, liver disease and obesity are all important conditions suffered by cats. Obesity is not only a common problem in pet cats, but causes a great deal of unnecessary suffering. I consider it to be a major animal-welfare issue that should not exist, because it is entirely preventable. Ageing is a natural, inevitable process experienced by cats who enjoy a long life, but can bring with it a range of problems and disabilities.

Cancer

Cancer is a very general term used to describe any kind of tumour that is found within or on a cat's body. A tumour is a mass of cells that occurs as a result of normal cells undergoing pointless and persistent division and proliferation. As every cell in a cat's body has the potential to initiate tumour growth, a cat may suffer from tumours of any tissue or body organ.

Tumours may be described as benign or malignant, depending on their appearance and the way in which they grow. Benign tumours are typically slow-growing, and do not usually become intimately associated with the surrounding tissues. They are normally less serious than the more aggressive malignant tumours, which are typically fast-growing, irregularly shaped masses of cells. These tend to infiltrate the tissues around them, and to spread to other distant body tissues and organs. Malignant tumours on the skin often ulcerate, bleed and become infected.

In the cat, almost one-third of all tumours are lymphomas. These are tumours that result from cancerous changes affecting certain cells of the immune system (lymphocytes). Lymphomas may affect just one part of a cat's body, or a number of different parts at the same time. They may also be associated with leukaemia, or abnormalities, in a cat's blood.

The other types of tumour that most commonly affect cats include the following:
- Skin tumours
- Soft-tissue tumours
- Breast tumours
- Mouth (oral) tumours
- Bone tumours
- Tumours of the digestive system

Causes

The vast majority of lymphomas in cats are caused by feline leukaemia virus infection (see pages 82–3), but the precise initial cause of other types of cancer is rarely – if ever – identified. Apparently normal cells may spontaneously initiate the development of tumours, or the tumours may be encouraged to develop under the influence of factors such as unidentified viruses, chemicals or radiation. Genetic and hormonal influences may also be involved in some cases of cancer.

It takes a change in behaviour of just one cell to create a tumour.

Is it serious?

All tumours, no matter how small, should be considered potentially serious until proven otherwise by a vet. Benign tumours are not usually fatal, but malignant tumours are invariably fatal if left untreated.

Cats at risk

Cancer is often thought of as only affecting older cats, but young cats can suffer from certain tumours.

Action

If you discover a lump or bump on your cat, or any other unusual change in his appearance, your vet should see him as soon as possible. Adopting a 'wait-and-see' approach may put your cat's life at risk.

Never ignore any other, non-specific symptoms of illness or debility that your cat shows. There is always a chance, especially if your cat is an older individual, that such symptoms may be associated with cancer. The longer a tumour remains untreated, the more likely it is to spread and the more difficult it will be to treat. The sooner it can be identified and its precise type diagnosed, the sooner your vet will be able to instigate any appropriate

---

COMMON SYMPTOMS

The symptoms that are associated with a tumour will depend on a range of factors, including its size and location, its interference with normal body processes and on whether it is benign or malignant.
- Some tumours, such as those affecting the skin or mouth, may be obvious at an early stage of their development; the existence of internal body tumours may not be detectable until they become more advanced.

treatment and the better the long-term outlook is likely to be.

Many cancers are diagnosed by vets during investigations into the possible causes of specific illness symptoms. For instance, a lame cat may turn out to be suffering from arthritis (see pages 42–3), but could have bone cancer. Typical means by which tumours may be identified include physical examination, X-ray and ultrasound investigations, blood tests and examinations using an endoscope (see pages 91–2).

If your vet confirms a tumour, he or she is likely to carry out further specific tests to identify its type, size, involvement with surrounding tissues and whether it has spread elsewhere in your cat's body. To do so, he or she may carry out further X-ray and ultrasound examinations, and take biopsies or other samples of the tumour (see page 92) for analysis by a pathologist.

Your vet may carry out the above investigations, or may refer your cat to a cancer specialist.

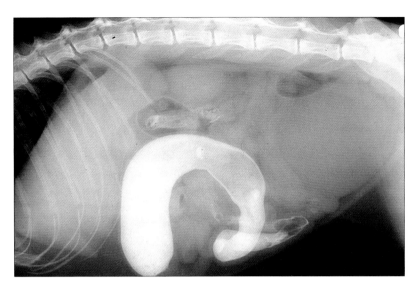

This is an X-ray of a cat's abdomen, taken after he had eaten a barium meal. The barium (white) has accumulated in a loop of small intestine because its normal passage is blocked by a tumour.

Treatment

Once your vet, or a specialist, has discovered all that he or she can about the tumour, any treatment options that may exist can be discussed. Our knowledge of how to treat tumours in cats is growing all the time, and options currently employed include the following:

Surgery • This may be undertaken to remove the tumour mass. Often large areas of tissue have to be removed in association with fairly small tumours, to reduce the risk of any tumour cells being left behind. The nature, extent and complexity of any surgical procedure will depend on the type of tumour present, on its size and degree of attachment to other tissues, and on its location.

Chemotherapy • This makes use of certain combinations of powerful drugs to help to kill tumour cells.

Radiotherapy • This is targeted at localized tumours, and is often carried out as part of a combined treatment regime that will also involve surgery. To reduce the side-effects of radiotherapy, a treatment course is normally split up into many doses.

Hyperthermia • This involves applying very high temperatures to a tumour in order to destroy the cells within it. The source of the heat is either ultrasound or electromagnetic radiation. This kind of therapy is often used in combination with a course of radiotherapy, and is most applicable to skin tumours.

Certain types of tumour respond best to individual treatments, or to combinations of therapies: your vet or a specialist will decide what is most appropriate for your cat.

Aftercare

At home, you must administer medicines to your cat and provide special care (see pages 98–111). Your vet will advise you on what to do.

Prevention

I would advise that your cat is vaccinated against feline leukaemia virus infection (see pages 82–3), the major cause of lymphomas in cats.

YOUR CAT'S FUTURE

No form of cancer therapy offers a guarantee of a permanent cure. If your cat has a serious tumour, the decision as to whether to go ahead with treatment, to let nature take its course, or to end his suffering painlessly through euthanasia (see pages 124–5) may be very difficult to make.

It is absolutely essential that you fully understand your cat's problem, and the kind of future that he may be able to have, with and without treatment. Listen carefully to your vet's advice, and discuss all the options available so that you can make the decision that is best for your cat.

Diabetes mellitus

This is a very complex condition, in which a cat is unable to control his blood-sugar (-glucose) levels. It affects up to one in 400 cats.

Causes

A cat's blood-glucose levels are controlled by the hormone insulin. This is produced by his pancreas, an organ lying close to his stomach that also produces some enzymes needed for digestion.

A cat with diabetes mellitus either suffers from a shortfall in the amount of insulin that his body needs, or produces enough insulin but his body tissues do not respond properly to its presence. The result is higher-than-normal blood levels of glucose in an affected individual.

The causes of diabetes mellitus in the cat are not well-understood, but may include failure of the pancreas to make sufficient insulin, or resistance of a cat's tissues to the effects of insulin that the pancreas produces (this may occur as a result of other hormonal conditions).

In addition, the long-term use of certain drugs – particularly certain female sex hormones commonly used to treat skin conditions such as miliary dermatitis (see pages 58–9) – may literally exhaust the ability of the pancreas to produce insulin.

Is it serious?

A cat who has untreated diabetes mellitus will – sooner or later – become depressed, vomit, breathe more rapidly than normal, stop passing any urine at all, and will eventually go into a coma and die.

Cats at risk

Diabetes mellitus appears to be most common in cats over six years old and in males, particularly those who have been neutered. Certain breeds may be more at risk than others, but evidence of this is still unclear. Obesity (see pages 76–7) is also considered to be a factor, although its precise role in this condition is not yet clear.

Action

If your cat exhibits any of the symptoms described, take him to your vet as soon as possible.

Many of the signs of diabetes mellitus are also common to other conditions, so your vet will consider the history of your cat's symptoms carefully and will then examine him thoroughly. He or she should carry out blood tests, and possibly urine tests (to look for glucose in the urine).

Treatment

Initially, your vet is likely to admit your cat as an in-patient, to try to stabilize his condition. If your cat is very ill, he will need intensive care. Before any form of treatment is started to help to control his

---

COMMON SYMPTOMS

An affected cat passes more urine than normal: this is because, when blood-glucose levels are too high, glucose is lost together with water through the kidneys.

Other typical symptoms may include the following:
• Increased thirst, due to the increased production of urine.
• An altered appetite: this is sometimes increased, but more commonly decreased.
• Weight loss
• Poor coat condition
• Lethargy
• Depression

---

condition in the long term, it is essential that you are aware of the responsibilities that you must take on in caring for your cat, and that your vet knows how much you are willing to do (see opposite, below).

The following are all common elements of therapy.

Treatment of the cause • This will be implemented if a specific cause (such as another hormonal condition) is identified.

Withdrawal of other drugs • Any drug treatment that could be a cause of the condition should be stopped as soon as possible.

Insulin given by injection • This must be carried out on a very regular schedule.

Urine samples • You may have to take these from your cat to test for the presence of glucose.

Dietary modification • There is no hard evidence supporting a particular dietary regime for diabetic cats, but the current view is that they may benefit from a high-fat, low-starch and low-fibre diet. In most cases, this means making no change to the normal diet, but your vet will give you precise advice for your cat. It is essential that his diet does not vary in consistency or in quantity from day to day. Every person who comes into contact with him must understand that he is not allowed any titbits, and that he has set mealtimes that are strictly enforced.

Exercise management • A diabetic cat must have a consistent daily level of exercise. Ideally, he should either be kept indoors permanently, or allowed access outside only in an enclosed garden or run (see page 40). This kind of management regime will

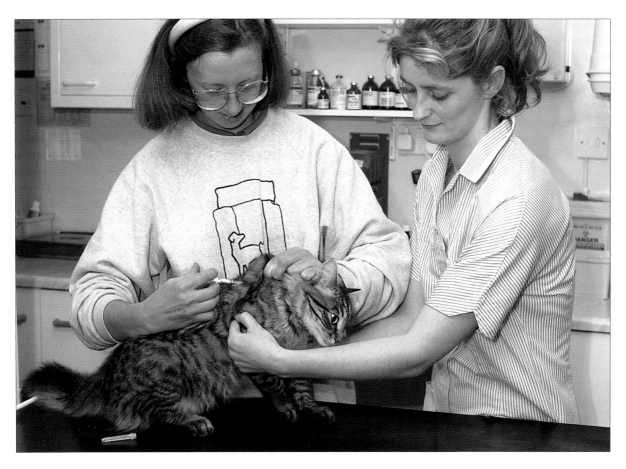

If your cat is diabetic, he is likely to need regular insulin injections at home. Your vet or a nurse may ask you to practise the technique on an orange!

not only help you to control his exercise, but will also allow you to monitor your cat and to obtain urine samples needed for regular glucose testing (special litter-trays should be available from your vet centre for this purpose).

Aftercare
Your vet will give you precise instructions about how to care for your cat at home. You must monitor your cat's condition very carefully (see pages 110–11), and will have to take him for regular check-ups.

If your cat is unwell in any way, or you are at all worried about him, contact your vet centre.

Prevention
The association between obesity and diabetes mellitus in cats is not fully understood, but the fact that

there seems to be a link is one of many good reasons why you should ensure that your cat does not become overweight. The best way to do this is to weigh him on a weekly basis (see pages 8–9): if your cat's weight begins to creep up, cut down his food accordingly.

CARING FOR A DIABETIC CAT

The following is a typical schedule carried out by an owner whose cat has diabetes mellitus.
• **Early morning:** Collect a urine sample and test it for glucose (once your cat has been stabilized on a set dose of insulin, urine tests may only be needed weekly).

• **30 minutes later:** Give morning feed (⅓ to ½ daily ration). Calculate how much insulin to inject, based on the urine test and food eaten.
• **5 minutes later:** Inject correct insulin dose under the skin.
• **8 hours later:** Give afternoon meal (½ to ⅔ daily ration).

Hyperthyroidism

This refers to a condition in which an affected cat has more thyroid hormone than normal circulating in his blood. It is the most common hormonal condition of the cat.

Causes

Most cases of hyperthyroidism in cats are caused by a form of benign cancer (see pages 68–9) involving one or both thyroid glands, which are positioned on either side of a cat's windpipe, or trachea.

Is it serious?

Persistently high levels of thyroid hormones in a cat's body cause severe symptoms, and may lead to other major conditions such as cardiomyopathy (see pages 34–5), so hyperthyroidism should be taken very seriously. However, despite its serious nature, this condition is treatable in most cases.

Cats at risk

Hyperthyroidism has been known to occur in cats of six years old, but most affected cats are over 10 years old. Males and females seem to be equally affected. There is some evidence that pure-bred cats may be less likely than cross-bred cats to suffer from this condition.

Action

If your cat shows any symptoms described, take him to your vet as soon as possible. Do not dismiss any of the symptoms (particularly behavioural changes) as the results of old age: let your vet be the judge.

Your vet will examine your cat thoroughly, and may be able to feel enlargement of one or both of his thyroid glands, although in many cases this is not possible. He or she is likely to carry out blood tests,

COMMON SYMPTOMS

Thyroid hormone influences the way in which many parts of a cat's body works, so the symptoms shown may vary considerably. The most consistent symptoms are weight loss and an

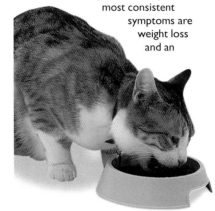

increased appetite, but additional symptoms may include the following:
• Behavioural changes: particularly hyperactivity, irritability and intolerance of heat.
• Increased thirst
• Poor coat condition
• Vomiting (see pages 26–7)
• Diarrhoea (see pages 32–3)
• A change in 'voice'
• A few cats in the advanced stages of hyperthyroidism may have a reduced appetite and be depressed and weak.

Many hyperthyroid cats have an increased appetite but actually lose weight. If you monitor your cat's food intake and weigh him regularly, you will spot these symptoms early.

and possibly also ECG, X-ray and ultrasound investigations (see pages 91–2). Thyroid scans, which involve the use of radioactive-marker substances, may be used at some specialist veterinary hospitals.

Treatment

In most cases of hyperthyroidism, the affected thyroid gland (or glands) will be removed surgically. Initially, however, your vet may treat your cat with anti-thyroid medicines and other drugs that are aimed at alleviating the effects of cardiomyopathy caused by the hyperthyroidism (see pages 34–5). The purpose of this is to get your cat into better physical condition before he undergoes surgery.

Anti-thyroid medicines will control the production of excessive amounts of thyroid hormones by a diseased gland. They have no effect on the underlying cause, and their long-term use is avoided if at all

possible because of their known side-effects (particularly adverse influences on bone marrow). The tablets also need to be given three times a day (see page 101), which is resented by most ill cats.

In some specialist veterinary hospitals, radioactive substances may be used in the treatment of hyperthyroid cats.

Many cats show a fairly dramatic improvement after treatment, but in some the condition recurs after two to three years.

Aftercare

You must keep your cat rested and confined indoors prior to surgery, and administer any prescribed medicines (see pages 101–2).

After surgery, your cat will be kept as an in-patient for a few days so that he can be monitored. You will then be told exactly how to nurse him during his convalescence (see also pages 98–111).

Ruptured diaphragm

The diaphragm is a sheet of muscle that separates the abdomen from the chest. It plays an important role in the mechanical process by which a cat sucks air into his lungs when he breathes in. If the diaphragm tears, it is said to have ruptured.

Causes

A ruptured diaphragm is most often suffered by a cat as a result of sudden, violent trauma, such as might occur in association with a collision with a vehicle or on impact after a nasty fall. Most diaphragm tears resulting from such injuries are triangular in shape.

Is it serious?

A ruptured diaphragm is a life-threatening condition.

Action

If your cat is involved in any kind of major accident, you may have to carry out emergency first aid (see pages 116–17). If he arrives home and is has laboured breathing, put

COMMON SYMPTOMS

The overall symptoms shown will depend on the combined effect of the injuries sustained. If your cat survives the initial accident, his abdominal organs may move forwards into his chest and will cause some amount of lung collapse as a result. The degree of collapse will be in line with the quantity of abdominal contents that can find their way through the ruptured diaphragm.
• Severe breathing difficulty is the most obvious symptom of a ruptured diaphragm.
• An affected cat is also likely to be lethargic.

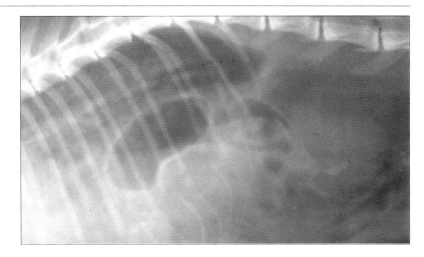

him in his carrying basket and then contact your vet centre urgently. Even if your cat does not seem very badly injured, you must still contact your vet centre immediately.

Your vet will tell you what to do, and may well ask you to bring your cat to the vet centre. He or she will examine your cat, and will listen very carefully to his chest with a stethoscope, and is also likely to carry out an X-ray investigation of his chest (see page 91).

Treatment

As well as a ruptured diaphragm your cat may have other injuries, and your vet will carry out any appropriate treatments in the order in which they are most needed. Your cat may be subjected to any or all of the following procedures:

Fluid therapy • Special fluids may be administered via an intravenous drip (see page 93).

Medicines • These may be given to counteract shock and relieve the pain.

Oxygen administration • This will be carried out (either via a mask, or in an oxygen tent) if your cat

In this X-ray picture of a cat lying on his side, a large 'bean-shaped' structure is obvious: this is a piece of bowel that contains air. It has been able to move from the cat's abdomen into his chest through a rupture in the diaphragm.

is experiencing such difficulty in breathing that he is unable to get enough oxygen into his blood.

Surgery • When your cat is in a suitable condition, your vet will operate to remove the abdominal contents from his chest and to replace them where they belong. He or she will then try to repair the diaphragm. The anaesthetic procedure required is complex and carries a significant risk that your cat may die but, as surgery is the only option, the potential benefits still outweigh the risks.

Aftercare

Your cat will be kept in for intensive care until your vet considers that he can return home. You may need to confine your cat to a cage at first, and (see page 106), and it may be many weeks before he is fit enough to venture outdoors again.

Liver disorders

The liver is one of a cat's major organs. It has many vital functions, including the production of most blood proteins, the conversion of the waste products of protein-processing into a substance that can be removed from the body by the kidneys, the processing and storage of carbohydrates and fats, the purification of the blood, and the production of bile to aid digestion.

A cat's liver may be affected by a number of conditions.

Causes

The following are liver conditions that are known to affect cats.

Hepatic lipidosis • This is the excess accumulation of fat within the liver. It may occur as a result of conditions such as diabetes mellitus (see pages 70–1) and obesity (see pages 76–7), or after starvation. However, in most severe cases the cause remains unknown: these so-called idiopathic cases generally occur in older animals who are stressed and have stopped eating. This condition is unusual in the UK but more common in the USA.

Cholangiohepatitis complex • This refers to a group of inflammatory disorders of the bile-producing parts of the liver. The condition is thought to be the most common liver disorder in cats in the UK, and often recurs in affected individuals. The cause is not known, but bacterial infection may be involved.

Toxic hepatopathy • Due to the way that his liver works, a cat cannot process some potentially toxic compounds quickly, and so is prone to being poisoned by the inappropriate use of certain drugs, such as aspirin. A cat who is suffering from this condition may go into sudden liver failure. Increased thyroid hormones resulting from hyperthyroidism (see page 72) may also have toxic effects on the liver.

Other causes • The liver may also be affected by other conditions. These include cancer, especially some forms of lymphoma (see pages 68–9), feline infectious peritonitis (see page 82) and developmental abnormalities that are present from birth.

Is it serious?

Any condition affecting the liver must be taken extremely seriously. Some cats who have certain liver conditions will respond to prompt treatment; others may die.

Action

If your cat exhibits the symptoms listed, or is in any way 'off-colour', take him to see your vet.

There is no simple test that can be carried out to identify a specific liver condition, so your vet will

---

COMMON SYMPTOMS

A cat who is suffering from a liver condition may be extremely ill, but symptoms are often vague. These may include the following:
• A reduced appetite or complete anorexia (refusal to eat)
• Depression
• Lethargy
• Weight loss
• Vomiting (see pages 26–7)
• Diarrhoea (see pages 32–3)
• Abdominal swelling
• Jaundice (this symptom is most obvious as a yellowing of the 'whites' of the eyes).

---

examine your cat, and may carry out blood and urine tests, and X-ray and ultrasound investigations. He or she may also sample and analyse fluid from the abdomen, and may in an exceptional case take biopsy samples of the liver (see page 92).

Your vet may resort to opening up your cat's abdomen surgically, to look directly at his liver, if other tests do not prove helpful.

Treatment

Treatment may include any or all of the following:

Intensive care • If your cat is very ill he will need intensive care, including fluids by intravenous drip (see page 93) and perhaps foods given by feeding tube.

Medication • Antibiotics may be needed if infection is suspected, and steroids (see page 97) may be given in a case of inflammatory liver disease.

Other treatment • Any specific treatments appropriate to an identified underlying cause will be implemented.

Dietary modification • The aim here is to reduce the build-up of waste products of protein-processing that occur in liver disease, which cause many of its symptoms. Your cat's diet should include easily digested carbohydrates (such as rice) to provide energy, and high-quality, easily digested protein (such as egg). Small amounts of food should be given frequently, with enough consumed to prevent weight loss: some cats may need force-feeding (see pages 104–5). Your vet will advise you about dietary changes, such as offering a prepared diet formulated for cats with liver conditions.

Anaemia

Anaemia is a symptom rather than a condition in its own right, and refers to a lower-than-normal number of red blood cells in a cat's blood. Each red cell contains a protein called haemoglobin: this gives the cell its colour and enables it to carry oxygen picked up at the lungs to other parts of the body.

Before birth, a cat's red blood cells are made in his bone marrow, liver and spleen, but, after birth, they are made only in the bone marrow. The rate at which new red cells are produced is influenced by the level of oxygen reaching the tissues. If the amount of oxygen that reaches the kidneys is too low, the kidneys produce a hormone that stimulates the bone marrow to produce more red blood cells.

Causes

There are a number of causes of anaemia, including the following:
• The reduced lifespan of red blood cells due to excessive breakdown: for instance, as a result of feline infectious anaemia (see above, right), abnormalities in the immune system or poisoning: for example, by paracetamol (see page 97).
• The loss of red blood cells due to bleeding or haemorrhaging (this may not be obvious: for instance,

---

FELINE INFECTIOUS ANAEMIA

In the UK, this condition is caused by an organism called *Haemobartonella felis*. This organism is parasitic on an affected cat's red blood cells, and causes their destruction or removal from the blood.

The infection can occur in any cat, although it generally affects those who are between one and three years

old. Currently, it is not known how the organism is transmitted.

Specific treatment using certain antibiotics is rarely completely successful, and many cats appear to become carriers of infection and may suffer from relapses. As many as one in four cats may die as a result of their infection with this organism.

---

low-grade, long-term internal bleeding into the digestive system may easily pass unnoticed).
• The reduced production of red blood cells from bone marrow, due to renal failure (see pages 64–5).
• Anaemia may occur in association with feline immunodeficiency virus (see pages 80–2) or feline leukaemia virus infection (see pages 82–3).

Is it serious?

All living tissues rely on red blood cells to supply oxygen to them, so anaemia is a very serious condition.

Cats at risk

All cats are at risk of anaemia.

Action

If your cat exhibits any of the symptoms described, keep him

quiet indoors and take him to your vet as soon as possible. If he is very lethargic and having problems in breathing, you must contact your vet centre immediately.

Your vet will examine your cat thoroughly and will carry out blood tests. Depending on the results of these, he or she may then undertake other procedures, such as X-ray investigations, endoscopy of your cat's digestive system, and even analysis of bone-marrow samples (see pages 91–2).

Treatment

Your vet will start treatment based on resolving the cause: for instance, stopping any bleeding or treating renal failure (see pages 64–5). He or she may also administer steroids (see page 97) to stimulate the bone marrow. In a severe case, a blood transfusion may also be necessary.

Aftercare

Until he has fully recovered, your cat must rest indoors. You will need to nurse him (see pages 98–111) and to administer prescribed medicines.

Prevention

Your cat should be vaccinated against feline leukaemia virus infection (see pages 82–3 and 85).

COMMON SYMPTOMS

The precise symptoms will depend on the severity of the anaemia, on the underlying cause and on the degree to which the cat's body has been able to compensate: for instance, by producing more red blood cells from his bone marrow. Typical symptoms may include the following:
• Pale gums

• Lethargy and weakness (these may not be spotted early on, as many owners do not know precisely how much activity their cats normally indulge in each day).
• Reduced appetite
• Weight loss
• Intolerance of the cold
• Rapid breathing on exertion

Obesity

Obesity is a disease associated with the accumulation of fat in a cat's body greater than is necessary for his body to function at its best. It is a very common condition.

Obesity may be linked with a number of other serious problems and conditions, including arthritis (see pages 42–3), diabetes mellitus (see pages 70–1) and liver disease: especially hepatic lipidosis (see page 74). It may result in breathing difficulties, heart and circulatory problems, an increased risk of suffering from infections and increased surgical risk.

Causes

The causes of obesity are complex, but the underlying problem is very straightforward. If, over a period of time, a cat's diet contains more energy (calories) than he burns up, his body will accumulate fat. If this imbalance remains uncorrected, he will become obese.

Owners do not deliberately encourage their cats to become obese, but many inadvertently do so. The following are some of the common mistakes made:
• Failing to adjust a cat's total food intake to his actual requirements, and ignoring the additional calories supplied by titbits. Although many cats seem to regulate their own food intake very accurately when offered free access to it, others do not.
• Believing that a large appetite is a sign of good health.
• Encouraging a cat to beg or to perform tricks, and then rewarding him with very palatable treats.
• Confining a cat indoors without adequate opportunities for exercise.
• Offering many different foods in the belief that this will prevent any nutritional 'inadequacies' in an individual product.
• Misinterpreting feeding guides on prepared foods (see opposite).

Other factors that may make a cat prone to obesity include his genetic make-up and neutering (castration and spaying).

Is it serious?

Many seriously obese cats have a miserable quality of life (most owners of formerly obese cats comment that their cats have gained a completely new lease of life as a result of losing weight).

There is also little doubt that uncorrected obesity can reduce an affected cat's life expectancy.

Cats at risk

All cats are at risk, but some experts believe that male, neutered cross-bred individuals are more likely to become obese.

Action

If you know that your cat is overweight, or you think that he may be, take him to see your vet – not next week, or next month, but today. Do not avoid taking him from embarrassment over being partly to blame. Obesity is not just an aesthetic problem, but a serious disease. If your cat is overweight he will be suffering unnecessarily, and you are the only person who can help him.

At your vet centre, your vet or a nurse will weigh your cat, and will examine him in order to assess the degree of obesity and to establish whether he is suffering from any other associated conditions. This may involve carrying out blood tests, and any other diagnostic procedures that prove necessary.

Treatment

Your vet will initiate any treatment needed to deal with any related conditions, and should then put together a tailor-made plan aimed at reducing your cat's weight in a controlled and scientific manner. Your input here is essential, as you will be the one to carry it out: unless you and your family are committed to your cat's slimming campaign, it is unlikely to be effective.
Dietary adjustment • In many good vet centres, highly trained veterinary nurses are in charge of creating individual weight-reduction programmes for obese cats. Although it may be possible

---

COMMON SYMPTOMS

These will depend on the degree of obesity and on any other conditions involved, but typical symptoms may include the following:
• An excess covering of fat over the ribs (if your cat is at his ideal weight, you should easily be able to feel his ribs through his skin; if you can see them, he is probably too thin).
• A flabby abdominal wall
• A waddling walk

• A large, pendulous flap of skin – containing fat – that dangles between the hindlegs.
• Lethargy
• Difficulty in jumping
• Becoming stuck in the cat flap!
It is generally accepted that – with a few exceptions – the ideal weight for the majority of healthy adult cats should be in the range of 3.5–4.5 kg (8–10 lb).

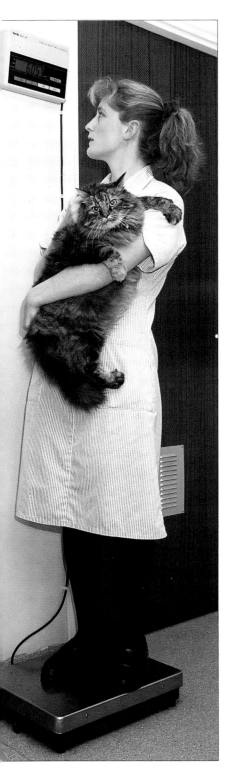

Your vet or nurse will wish to examine and weigh your cat on a regular basis, in order to check on his progress.

CAT-FOOD FEEDING GUIDES

The feeding guide on a cat-food label gives recommendations, but your cat will be like no other when it comes to his food. You will need to adjust the amount that you offer him to match his personal requirements.

If you change him to a new food, begin by mixing a little of this with some of the old food to prevent a digestive upset, and then gradually increase the proportion of the new food. After a day or two, offer your cat a daily amount based on the feeding guide on the product label. Weigh your cat every week, and adjust his food as necessary.

simply to cut down your cat's current diet, doing so may lead to nutritional imbalances. What is more, his current feeding regime may have contributed to his obesity in the first place. As a result, it is likely that your vet or nurse will base your cat's new feeding regime on a prepared low-calorie diet (see page 105).

Exercise management • In theory, increased physical activity can help weight reduction in cats, but this can be very difficult to achieve in practice. The only options here are to increase the amount of time that you spend playing with your cat, or, if at the moment he is confined indoors, you could consider giving him free access outdoors or restricted access to an outdoor enclosure or enclosed garden.

Your vet or nurse will monitor your cat's progress very carefully and, when he reaches his ideal weight, will offer you further dietary and exercise advice aimed at keeping him that way in the long term. You will need to take your cat back to see your nurse as advised: this is likely to be at two-week intervals, or more frequently in the initial stages. Many vet centres now run slimming clinics for cats.

Prevention

The most important way to prevent obesity is to plan a sensible and appropriate feeding regime for your cat right from the start. Rather than attempting to make nutritional decisions unaided, you should ask for advice from someone trained in nutrition, such as your vet or a veterinary nurse.

If you have a kitten, you should weigh him regularly. Your vet or a veterinary nurse should be happy to create a growth chart for your kitten, for comparison with that of a normal kitten: this will reveal whether you are inadvertently making any feeding mistakes.

Even if your cat is an adult, you should weigh him once a week. This is especially important if you change his diet, or if his lifestyle alters in any way: for instance, if he is confined due to illness. By doing this, you can fine-tune the amount that you feed: if you notice a slight drop in your cat's weight, you can increase his food slightly; if he puts on weight, cut back his food a little. It really is that simple.

WARNING

If at any stage during his slimming campaign – but particularly during the initial stages – your cat refuses to eat or is in any way unwell, you must contact your vet centre.

Growing old (ageing)

Cats are now living longer than ever before. If the stories are to be believed, some cats have survived into their thirties, but a good innings for a cat is perhaps nearer to 15 years.

Neutered cats generally tend to live longer than those who have not been spayed or castrated. This may be because entire (unneutered) cats roam more and, as a result, may be more prone to injury associated with exposure to environmental hazards. In general, cross-bred cats and those of very mixed origins are thought to have a longer life-expectancy than pure-bred cats.

A cat's body is a remarkable creation. It is able to repair itself and has built-in spare parts: for instance, a cat has two kidneys but actually needs only part of one kidney to stay healthy (see page 64). Inevitably, however, the years take their toll, and like humans, cats experience numerous bodily changes associated with ageing.

You can help to improve your cat's chances of enjoying a long life by providing him with a lifetime of good nutrition, exercise and healthcare, together with special care during the last third of his expected life – his golden years.

The ageing changes

The following are just some of the common problems that may be faced by an older cat:
• Decreased sensitivity to thirst, leading to possible dehydration.
• Decreased body-temperature control, leading to a much-reduced tolerance of heat and cold.
• A shallow sleep pattern, resulting in irritability.
• Decreased sensitivity of hearing, sight, taste and smell.

• Greater susceptibility to infection
• Periodontal disease and tooth loss (see pages 22–4).
• Decreased saliva production and swallowing difficulties.
• Mouth ulcers
• Digestive upsets, due to decreases in the ability of the stomach and intestines to digest food.
• Arthritis (see pages 42–3) and joint stiffness
• Skin abnormalities, such as coat dullness, alopecia (see pages 48–9), and also abnormally shaped and brittle claws.
• Decreased kidney and liver function (see pages 64–5 and 74).
• Cancer (see pages 68–9)
• Muscle weakness
• Weaker and more brittle bones
• High blood pressure
• Anaemia (see page 75)
• Breathing becomes less efficient at delivering oxygen to the blood, because the lungs become less flexible and the muscles involved in breathing weaken. This may contribute to problems such as tiredness on exercise, and altered behaviour associated with senility.
• Decreased numbers of cells in the brain are thought to lead to slow reaction times, partial memory loss, irritability and disorientation. The first sign of senility is often the loss of normal toileting habits.

Action

Providing your cat with a good diet, appropriate levels of exercise, a stimulating lifestyle and good healthcare from his kittenhood will make sure that he approaches old age in the best possible shape. From his tenth birthday onwards (see below), you should pay particular attention to the following:

Diet • An older cat may benefit from the following changes to his dietary regime:
• Less calories when he becomes less active. You should weigh your cat regularly and, if his weight begins to creep up, cut back his food accordingly.
• A more palatable diet (for example, of warmed, moist foods), because of his decreased senses of smell and taste.
• Avoidance of excess protein, phosphorus and sodium, increased amounts of vitamins A, B1, B6, B12 and E, and extra unsaturated fatty acids and zinc are nutritional modifications considered appropriate for older cats. As yet, there are no prepared foods that are available specifically for older cats (in the UK), so for now the best you can do is to ensure that you are feeding your cat a diet based on

PHYSICAL CHANGES IN AN OLDER CAT

Ageing changes take place a great deal more rapidly in a cat than they do in a person. In many ways, a cat's body at one year old is considered to be in a similar condition to that of a 16-year-old child. By two years old, he is more like a 21-year-old person. Each successive year for a cat is equivalent to four human years: for example, a nine-year-old cat has an equivalent human age of 49 years.

Although it is impossible to specify a precise age, some experts believe that most cats should be considered geriatric from a medical point of view when they reach the age of 10.

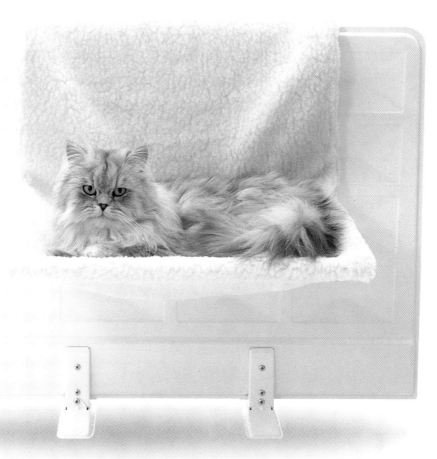

high-quality prepared foods suitable for adult cats. Your vet will keep you up to date with any new developments.

• Older cats are less tolerant of sudden diet changes, so make any alterations slowly. .

Health-checks • By carrying out regular health-checks on your cat (see pages 8–9) you will be much more likely to notice early symptoms of some common diseases to affect older cats, such as arthritis (see pages 42–3) and cancer (see pages 68–9).

Monitoring • Keep a close watch on your cat's urine and faeces by encouraging him to use a litter-tray if he does not do so already, and monitor his water intake for any obvious changes. You should pay particular attention to any changes in your cat's behaviour: no matter how subtle, they may be significant. If problems in an older cat are identified in their early stages, much can be done to tackle them. Anaesthetics (see pages 94–5) are now safer than they have ever been, and it is not uncommon for cats in their late teens or twenties to undergo major surgery successfully.

Preventive healthcare • Continue with intestinal- and skin-parasite prevention (see pages 28–9 and 54–8). Your vet should examine your cat at least twice a year: one opportunity for this will be when he is given his annual booster vaccination (see page 85).

Grooming • You should continue to groom your cat regularly, in order to maintain optimum coat and skin health (see page 51). Grooming can also be extremely therapeutic for cats who have been used to it from a young age.

A soft fleece cat bed that is designed to be hung over a radiator will be very warm and comfortable for an old cat.

Dental care • Periodontal disease is a major problem in older cats, so routine tooth-brushing should be continued in those who will accept it (see pages 22–4).

Exercise • Older cats – even those with arthritis (see pages 42–3) – need regular exercise to maintain muscle bulk and strength. Exercise also provides mental stimulation and encourages bowel function. Even if your older cat stays indoors, play with him and do not let him sleep for hours at a time.

Your vet or a nurse will help you to evaluate your cat's lifestyle. Many vet centres run clinics to monitor the health of older cats: on your cat's tenth birthday, sign him up!

Major infectious diseases

All cats are vulnerable to a number of infectious diseases. These are caused by certain microscopic organisms – particularly viruses – that may be passed on from one infected cat to other healthy ones. The specific infectious diseases to which your cat may be exposed will depend on where you live, as well as on his lifestyle. For instance, if he meets many unfamiliar cats, or visits places that they frequent, he will be more susceptible to infections than a house cat.

The following are the major infectious diseases that may affect cats. (For information on feline viral upper-respiratory-tract disease, or cat 'flu, see pages 38–9.)

Feline chlamydiosis

Causes

This disease is caused by a feline strain of a very specialized type of bacteria called *Chlamydia psittaci*, which causes conjunctivitis (see pages 12–14). The infection is most common in kittens between five weeks and nine months old; often a whole litter of kittens may be affected at the same time.

A healthy cat is most likely to pick up the disease through direct contact with discharge from the eyes or nose of an infected cat, although the organism may survive away from a cat for as long as three days. The incubation period is about 14 days. Initially only one eye may be affected, but the other usually becomes involved one to three weeks later.

Common symptoms

If left untreated, severe symptoms of conjunctivitis (see pages 12–14) normally resolve over about three to four weeks. However, milder symptoms may persist for months, and apparently recovered cats may be contagious for up to 18 months.

Natural immunity following infection is fairly shortlived, and previously affected cats may have recurrent bouts of chlamydiosis, especially if they live with other cats in which the organism is able to circulate freely.

Despite their symptoms, most cats continue to eat and remain otherwise well. The organism can also infect a cat's reproductive and digestive systems, although such infections usually go unnoticed.

Treatment

This normally involves antibiotics being given by mouth, and frequent use of antibiotic eye ointments.

Prevention

Vaccination against this disease is available (see page 85), and is recommended particularly for cats who are exposed to environments in which chlamydiosis is, or has in the past been, a problem.

Feline immunodeficiency virus infection

In 1982, several cats in a colony in California became ill. Their symptoms varied, but included diarrhoea, nasal discharge and inflamed gums, and it seemed that their main problem was an inability to fight off infections: a condition called immunosuppression.

Feline leukaemia virus infection had been discovered 18 years before (see pages 82–3) and was known to cause immunosuppression, so this quickly became the prime suspect. It was the right virus family, but the wrong relative: none of the cats was infected with this virus. In 1986, after an extensive investigation, experts identified the cause as a virus previously unknown to science: feline immunodeficiency virus (FIV). FIV belongs to a group of viruses called 'retroviruses'. Other members of this group include FeLV (see pages 82–3), HIV (the cause of human AIDS) and other viruses that affect sheep, cattle and horses.

Since that time, scientists have found evidence of FIV infection in old blood samples from pet cats dating back to the late 1960s. In fact, wherever in the world anyone has looked for it, FIV has been found, and it is thought likely that the virus has existed for centuries.

FIV, which is related to HIV, appears only to be able to infect wild or pet cats. Up to one in 20 apparently healthy cats, and one in five 'ill' pet cats may be infected.

Causes

Scientists do not yet have all the answers about how FIV is spread, but they believe that the main

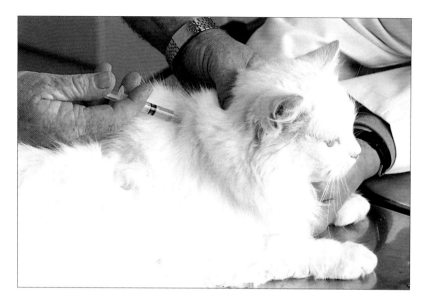

Routine vaccinations against many of the infectious diseases of cats are given by injection. Reactions to vaccinations are rare, but you should keep your cat indoors to observe him for 24 hours.

skin disorders (see pages 48–9) and anaemia (see page 75). Infection with FIV is diagnosed by means of a specific blood test.

Cats at risk

Symptoms associated with FIV infection seem to be more common in male, non-pedigree cats, in those who roam freely outdoors and in those between six and 10 years old.

Treatment

There is currently no specific treatment available for infection with FIV. Many of the anti-viral drugs used against HIV in people have been shown experimentally to be effective against FIV, but further tests are needed on the long-term use of these drugs in cats. For this reason, it is unlikely that they will be available in the near future.

method of transmission is by the injection of FIV in saliva when a cat is bitten by another infected cat. For the infection to be passed on, substantial quantities of the virus need to be injected in this way.

Outside the body, the virus is quickly destroyed and the spread of infection in confined groups of cats that do not fight is rare.

Common symptoms

About five weeks after infection, some – but not all – cats may be a little off-colour for several days, with a raised temperature. Most will also develop swollen glands all over their bodies that may stay swollen for many months. For the majority of cats, there then follows a period lasting for several months or even years when nothing further appears to happen.

When further symptoms do develop, they are generally the result of other recurrent infections or diseases – such as gingivitis-stomatitis (see pages 24–5) or rhinitis (see pages 40–1) – that eventually become permanent because FIV has suppressed the

affected cat's normal protective immune response to them.

Every FIV-infected cat's personal cocktail of symptoms will vary to some degree, but these may include lethargy, weight loss, conjunctivitis (see pages 12–14), a nasal discharge, gingivitis-stomatitis (see pages 24–5), diarrhoea (see pages 32–3),

IF YOUR CAT HAS FIV INFECTION

If your cat is diagnosed as having an FIV infection, there are a number of important further steps that you should consider taking, as follows:
• Ask your vet to blood-test any other cats that you have, in order to check whether they are also infected (this may not be conclusive, however, as some infected cats may come up clear on such tests).
• Provided that they do not fight, you can keep infected and non-infected cats together without any great risk of the infection being passed on. However, it is a good idea to feed the cats separately.
• If you keep a breeding colony, you should separate infected and non-infected cats as a precaution.

• Minimize contact with other strange cats to reduce the chances of your cat picking up any other infections and passing on FIV. If your cat is a known fighter, you should keep him indoors or give him restricted access outdoors in a fully enclosed garden or a suitable cage (see page 40).
• Be diligent about preventive-healthcare measures: keep your cat up to date with routine vaccinations (see page 85), carry out a thorough worming and flea-prevention campaign (see pages 28–9 and 56), offer him the highest-quality diet you can afford and groom him regularly.
• If your cat suddenly becomes ill in any way, contact your vet centre as soon as possible.

If your cat is diagnosed as having an FIV infection, your vet may be able to control the early symptoms with antibiotics and steroids (see pages 96–7), and by making dietary alterations. Long-term use of evening primrose oil may also help some cats.

The future for an FIV-infected cat will depend on when the diagnosis is made. If the cat is apparently healthy and in the early stages of the disease, it may be several years before serious symptoms develop.

At first, there is generally a good response to symptomatic treatment, but the symptoms usually become more and more difficult to treat, and other problems often develop.

By this stage, many cats have such a poor quality of life that, sadly, euthanasia is in their best interests (see pages 124–5).

Prevention

Unfortunately, the only foolproof way of preventing your cat from becoming infected with FIV is to make sure that he never meets another cat. A good compromise is to keep him in at night. Neutering will reduce a male cat's wanderings and his chances of being involved in sexually motivated fights.

There is currently no vaccine against FIV, and research scientists face many problems: for instance, the disease appears to have many strains, so a vaccine for one strain may be useless against another. It is unlikely that a vaccine will be developed for some years yet.

Feline infectious peritonitis

Causes

This condition is caused by strains of a virus called feline coronavirus. A healthy cat may pick these up via contact with the faeces or saliva of infected cats, before those cats show symptoms. At the time when most infected cats do develop symptoms of FIP, they are not contagious.

The outcome of infection will depend on many factors, including the precise strain and dose of the virus, the cat's age and the state of his immune system. He may fight off the infection and recover but, if his immune-system response is not sufficiently strong, the virus will spread around his body.

Common symptoms

The strength of a cat's immune-system response may determine whether he suffers from so-called 'wet' or 'dry' FIP. These are two extremes of a range of symptoms. Initial symptoms of both include a reduced appetite and lethargy.

If a cat goes on to suffer from 'wet' FIP, further symptoms will develop rapidly over just a few weeks, and will include abdominal swelling, fever, depression, weight loss and anaemia (see page 75). The chest may also fill with fluid, causing breathing difficulties.

Symptoms of 'dry' FIP take longer to appear, and are associated with development of inflammatory growths. Most commonly, these affect the liver, kidneys, brain and eyes; symptoms usually include weight loss, depression and fever.

Treatment

There is currently no specific treatment or vaccine for FIP. Most cats die as a result of infection.

Feline leukaemia virus infection

First discovered in 1964, feline leukaemia virus, or FeLV as it is better-known, is now considered to be one of the most significant causes of feline disease in the UK. Seven out of 10 cats are thought likely to come into contact with FeLV at some point in their lives, and – sooner or later – the infection is likely to result in the death of three out of 10 of them.

FeLV has been found in every country in which anyone has looked for it. In the UK, experts believe that as many as one in 20 apparently healthy cats living in urban or suburban environments may be permanently infected.

Causes

FeLV is highly infectious. The virus is present in the saliva, urine, blood, milk, respiratory mucus and faeces of permanently infected cats.

Saliva is the most common source of infection, and the virus can be passed on by regular close contact and by bite wounds (see pages 60–1). Kittens can pick up FeLV infection from their mothers, either before they are born, via their placentas, or via her milk.

There are three outcomes for an infected cat, depending on his age, on the response of his immune system and on the dose of virus that he has received.

• A cat may successfully fight off the infection and become naturally immune to re-infection. This is generally the rule in older cats.

• A cat may be completely overwhelmed by the virus. His immune system is unable to cope, and a permanent FeLV infection is the result. He will become a 'virus factory', making and then exporting virus particles to the outside world from within his body. In general, this is the expected result in about three out of every 10 cats exposed to the virus, and may be the norm in infections of unborn kittens and those less than eight weeks old. The majority of these infected kittens and cats will die within three-and-a-half years. The most common causes of death from FeLV result from immunosuppression (reduced immunity to other diseases), cancer – notably lymphomas (see pages 68–9) – and anaemia (see page 75).

• A cat's immune system may attack the virus, but may be unable to beat it off completely. Some virus will then remain inside his body, but – given enough time – he may still manage to eliminate it. If not, he may go on to suffer from FeLV-related tumours.

Cats at risk

All cats are at risk, and most will come into contact with the virus at least once in their lives. However, whether this leads on to serious disease, and ultimately death, depends on a number of factors, such as the age of the cat involved.

Common symptoms

There are no specific symptoms of this disease. A cat who is fighting the initial infection may simply appear off-colour, and in most cases the original infection will probably go unnoticed by owners.

Many signs of more advanced disease are also generally rather non-specific. As one of the main

---

IF YOUR CAT HAS FeLV

If your cat is diagnosed with FeLV infection, bear in mind the following:

• The diagnosis may not necessarily mean that your cat is permanently infected with FeLV and fatally ill. He may have only just been infected and, although he is fighting the virus, may not yet have eliminated it. This initial test may even have given a misleading result, so try not to panic. Your vet will wish to carry out further tests to clarify the situation.

• If you own other cats, your vet will tell you what to do. For instance, he or she is likely to suggest that your other cats are blood-tested.

• If your cat is confirmed as being permanently infected, you should only allow him access outdoors in a cat-proof garden or in an enclosed outdoor cage, to prevent him from passing on the infection.

• If your cat is female, you must not breed from her, as all her kittens will be infected with the virus.

• You are extremely unlikely to carry FeLV from your house to another house, so you do not need to avoid visiting cat-owning friends, and they can visit you and your cat.

• Be diligent about preventive-healthcare measures that you carry out for your cat: undertake regular worming and flea-prevention procedures (see pages 28–9 and 54–6), offer your cat the highest-quality diet that you are able to afford, keep him up to date with his routine vaccinations (see page 85), and groom him thoroughly on a regular and frequent basis.

• If your cat suddenly becomes ill in any way, contact your vet centre as soon as possible.

---

effects of permanent FeLV infection is a damping down of the immune system (immunosuppression), the actual symptoms are often those of other infections and diseases to which FeLV has made the cat prone.

The most common symptoms that are associated with permanent FeLV infection include weight loss, fever, conjunctivitis (see pages 12–14), mouth ulcers and gingivitis (see pages 24–5), vomiting (see pages 26–7), diarrhoea (see pages 32–3), and anaemia (see page 75), but there are many others. As the incubation period for FeLV-related diseases can be very long, these symptoms may appear months or years after infection.

A permanently infected cat may look completely healthy during the incubation period, yet all the time he will be pumping out the virus. Infection is diagnosed by a blood test. If this test is positive, it may be repeated some weeks later.

Treatment

There are no specific drugs available to treat FeLV infection. Sick, permanently infected cats can only be treated symptomatically in an attempt to make them feel more comfortable.

Prevention

Two vaccines are available in the UK (if you live outside the UK, ask at your vet centre for advice). The primary course for either vaccine is two injections, three to four weeks apart. Normally, an annual booster is all that is required from then on. Both vaccines are for kittens over nine weeks old. They can be given at the same times as other routine vaccinations (see page 85).

Remember that your cat may appear healthy, but could already be permanently infected. In this case vaccination will obviously be pointless, so your vet may test your cat for the virus first.

Feline panleucopenia (Feline infectious enteritis)

This condition was the first feline disease shown to be caused by a virus. It is a highly infectious disease that may affect any kind of cat, including lions, tigers and leopards, as well as other animals such as mink, ferret and racoon.

The virus is known for its ability to survive in the environment: it is resistant to heat as well as to many disinfectants, and can persist in contaminated premises for months.

Causes

Any cat of any age may become infected, but panleucopenia is usually a disease of young kittens. Infected cats will disseminate the virus that is responsible for this disease mainly in their faeces, but also in their saliva, urine, vomit and blood. In most cases, a cat becomes infected through direct contact with another cat who is infected, or through exposure to contaminated objects or environments.

Once established inside a cat's body, the virus heads for those parts that contain rapidly dividing cells, such as the bone marrow and the intestinal wall. In the case of a pregnant female cat, the virus may also infect her unborn kittens.

Common symptoms

In some cats there are few – if any – symptoms, but other infected cats may die suddenly. The incubation period is normally two to 10 days, and the first symptoms are fever, a reduced appetite, vomiting and lethargy. If a cat survives this stage, he may develop profuse watery diarrhoea within two to three days.

Unborn kittens infected at a late stage of pregnancy may develop symptoms associated with brain damage – such as lack of co-ordination – at a few weeks old.

Treatment

There is no specific treatment, and cats suffering from panleucopenia need intensive nursing care in total isolation from any other cats.

Some cats survive infection, but their convalescence usually takes several weeks, during which time they are prone to other infections because their immune defences have been so badly damaged. Those cats who do recover are thought to develop a lifelong immunity to re-infection with this virus.

Prevention

Kittens and older cats should be vaccinated against panleucopenia (see opposite).

Rabies

Rabies is a virus that can infect all mammals, and causes disease by affecting the central nervous system. The virus is found in all continents except Australasia and Antarctica but, due to geographical barriers and quarantine measures, certain countries – such as the UK – are currently thought to be free of it.

In some parts of the world, such as mainland Europe, the USA and Canada, the rabies virus mainly circulates among wild-animal species, but in other regions, such as Asia and Africa, over 95 per cent of cases occur in domestic dogs.

Causes

Rabies is nearly always transmitted by bite, as the virus is present in the saliva of infected animals and is not able to penetrate through intact skin. The incubation period is usually 15 to 25 days, but may be up to two months.

Common symptoms

The first symptoms are generally associated with subtle changes in temperament, and excessive licking and/or chewing at the initial bite wound. This may only last for one day. A quiet cat may become more alert, restless and interactive, whereas a friendly individual may become aggressive or depressed and withdrawn.

An infected cat may show a lack of appetite, or he may appear to be ravenous. He will gradually become more nervous, agitated and irritable, and may be vicious and uncoordinated in his movements. This so-called 'furious' stage of a rabies infection may last for up to a week, but some cats will progress from the initial symptoms straight to a state of paralysis, seizures, coma and death.

Treatment

There is no treatment currently available for rabies.

Prevention

Vaccines against the rabies virus are available, but in the UK these will only be administered to cats due to be exported, or who are entering quarantine. In countries in which rabies is a potential problem, cats should be vaccinated against the virus on a routine basis.

Preventing major infectious diseases

When a cat's body is invaded by a disease-causing organism such as a virus, his immune system should react to try to destroy it.

However, the organisms that cause some infectious diseases may be so quick to damage vital body organs and structures that the immune system cannot respond sufficiently fast to prevent critical illness or death. Alternatively, the immune system may be put out of action by the initial infection.

Vaccination

Vaccination improves the speed and effectiveness of a cat's immune-system response to a particular infection, by stimulating it through exposure to harmless amounts of an organism before the cat encounters it for real. Failure to keep up with your cat's vaccinations may put his life at risk.

Routine vaccinations are an essential component of your cat's preventive-healthcare plan (see also page 113).

NOTES ON VACCINATION

• Your vet or a veterinary nurse should give you a special record card containing details of any vaccinations that have been administered to your cat. You should keep this in a safe place with your cat's other medical records, and expect to be asked to produce it when you book him into a cattery or at any time by your vet.
• Obvious reactions to vaccinations are unusual, but some individuals may be a little quieter than normal for 24 hours. If you think that your cat has reacted badly to a vaccination, contact your vet centre immediately.
• Vaccinations do not give guaranteed protection from the major infectious diseases, but it is rare for a cat not to respond as expected to them.
• The vaccination needs of cats may vary from area to area, so discuss your cat's needs with your vet.

The exact timing of vaccinations will depend on the products used by your vet centre and the current vaccination recommendations in your region or country.

For the first few weeks of his life, while his own immune system is developing, a kitten should be protected from the major infectious diseases by consuming antibodies in his mother's first milk. He will also have gained some protection through the transfer of antibodies via his placenta. The queen should have produced these antibodies as a result of her own vaccinations, or through surviving natural infection. The protection obtained from these so-called maternal antibodies will wane as the kitten grows older, and will normally have disappeared altogether by the time that he is 12 weeks old.

In the UK, a typical vaccination regime may be as follows:

At nine weeks • Vaccination against feline herpesvirus and calicivirus, the viruses that cause cat 'flu (see pages 38–9), and feline leukaemia virus infection. These vaccinations may be administered as one injection, or the vaccination against FeLV may be given separately.

At 12 weeks • A repeat of the above vaccinations. A kitten should not go outdoors or be introduced to other cats (other than those with whom he lives) until seven to 10 days after this vaccination.

At 15 months • A repeat of the vaccination(s) given at 12 weeks. From this point onwards, the same vaccinations will be given at 12-monthly intervals, and are generally referred to as boosters.

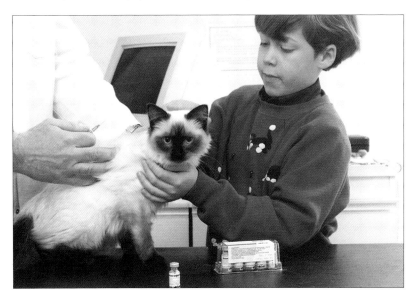

Vet centres and procedures

A good vet centre will offer you much more than just emergency medical care for your cat. This section offers practical advice on choosing and using your vet centre, and includes background information on some of the most common veterinary procedures that your cat may experience while he is there.

Your cat's health service

If your cat is injured or becomes ill, you will want the best medical attention for him. It is comforting to know that veterinary services are available 24 hours a day, 365 days a year from most vet centres. Even those that do not provide out-of-hours services themselves should make sure that the needs of their patients are properly catered for in an emergency.

The staff at your vet centre will not only treat your cat when he is unwell, but will be a mine of useful information about cat care. For your cat's sake, you should make good use of them. Ideally, you should register at a centre before you even obtain your cat, as the staff will be able to give you plenty of practical tips to help you to plan for his arrival.

They should also provide you with a range of healthcare services aimed at keeping your cat healthy. These so-called preventive-medicine services include parasite control, dietary advice, dental care and vaccination.

VETERINARY PROFESSIONALS
A number of key people play a part in the day-to-day work of a typical vet centre, and are all part of your cat's veterinary team.

Veterinary surgeons (Vets)
The vet who cares for your cat may not only be his physician but much more besides, including his personal surgeon, dentist, anaesthetist, pharmacist and perhaps even his psychiatrist! A large vet centre may have a number of vets working in it.

Many of the routine tasks that were formerly undertaken by vets are now being made the responsibility of the veterinary nurses at some centres, so that the vets can concentrate on more specialist work. Every vet is qualified to treat all kinds of animals – great and small – but some vets go on to take further qualifications in specific areas of veterinary work, such as dermatology or orthopaedics.

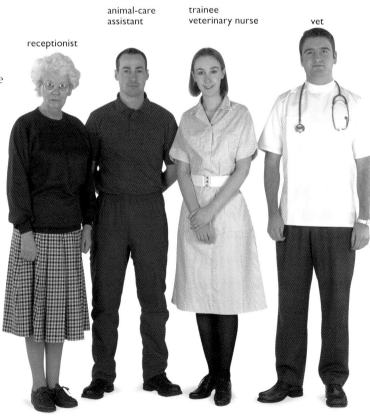

receptionist

animal-care assistant

trainee veterinary nurse

vet

Veterinary nurses

Skilled and highly trained veterinary nurses are, in my experience, the backbone of many vet centres. Just a few of their many responsibilities may include running the operating theatre, assisting vets with diagnostic, surgical and medical procedures, looking after in-patients, running the drugs dispensary, carrying out laboratory tests and organizing special clinics. Nurses may also perform some medical treatments and minor surgical procedures, under the guidance of a vet.

Animal-care assistants

Unqualified, but nevertheless very caring, animal-care assistants may be employed to reduce the workload of the veterinary nurses. Feeding in-patients, exercising them and cleaning up after them are all typical duties.

Receptionist

The receptionist is normally responsible for booking appointments, handling enquiries, collecting fees and generally ensuring that clients are looked after.

CHARITY CLINICS

In some areas, veterinary services are offered free, by animal charities, to pet-owners who are on some forms of state welfare. In the UK, for instance, the People's Dispensary for Sick Animals has over 40 clinics spread throughout the country. These clinics are run on public donations, and, in my view, those who use them should be prepared to help with fund-raising.

A dedicated receptionist should be adequately trained to offer basic advice about animal healthcare, but should not be expected to answer more serious medical queries.

Centre manager

A well-run vet centre can invest in new staff, facilities and equipment to ensure an ever-better service for both clients and patients. Some vet centres employ a centre manager, whose responsibilities will include the smooth running of the centre, the processing of accounts and the handling of client queries.

Other staff

Many vet centres also rely on the help of a number of other full-time or part-time staff, including cleaners and handymen. You may never see them, but if your cat ever has to stay in at your centre he will no doubt get to know them briefly, if only for a cuddle!

TYPES OF VET CENTRE

Some vet centres have the facilities and staff to treat animals of any sort – large or small– including horses, farm stock, dogs, cats and other pet animals; others concentrate solely on the care of pets, including the more exotic varieties such as reptiles.

Vet centres may also be called clinics, surgeries or practices, and the largest and best-equipped centres are sometimes called veterinary hospitals. In contrast, the smallest vet centres may have only basic equipment and facilities, and may be open to their clients for just a few hours a day. Between these two extremes are vet centres of all sizes.

vet (centre owner)   head veterinary nurse   veterinary nurse   centre manager

Get to know your cat's veterinary team. As well as making sure that both you and he are well looked after, the staff at a good centre will be a mine of useful information on every aspect of cat care.

CHOOSING A VET CENTRE

Research shows that most people simply use the vet centres that are nearest to their homes, although, as you will have discovered in the previous pages, not all vet centres are the same. The centre that is geographically most convenient to you may turn out to be the one best-suited to your needs, but do not simply assume that this is the case. Investigate the alternatives – if any exist – by following the steps outlined here.

If possible, you should make your initial decision well before you even collect your cat, so that you can benefit from all the advice available from the centre as you prepare to become a cat-owner.

What to do first

• Look in your local business telephone directory for vet centres, and make a list of all those that are within 20 to 30 minutes' drive – this is the furthest you should need to travel in an emergency.

A typical vet centre

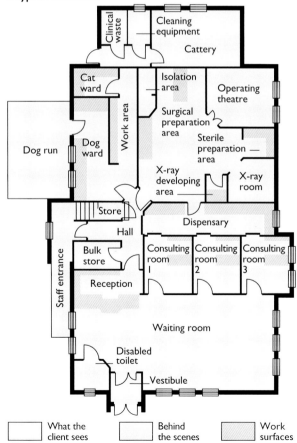

• Make a quick, unannounced visit to all the centres on your shortlist. On each visit, take note of the difficulty of the journey, the ease of access to the premises and parking facilities, the state of repair of the premises, the cleanliness of the waiting room and reception area, and the appearance and attitude of the receptionist.
• Ask for information about the vet centre, including details of services offered to cat-owners, the centre's opening times and the fees charged (many good centres will produce a brochure). Find out whether it would be possible to arrange a tour of the centre. If you can, wait about looking at the notice-board long enough to see how other clients are handled.

What to do next

• Speak to cat-owning friends to obtain their opinions of the centres on your initial list.
• Armed with the information that you have obtained on each centre, and with your friends' views in mind, prepare a new shortlist. You should not even consider a centre that is not prepared to give you a guided tour of their facilities. What must they have to hide? All good centres will be happy to give you a guided tour, although this may have to be outside normal working hours for obvious reasons. Some centres now run regular open days to enable current and prospective clients to see behind the scenes.
• Arrange to view the centres that you have shortlisted. If possible, go as a family or take a friend, as second opinions are always valuable. While you are there, try to meet some of the veterinary staff, and take note of their appearance and friendliness.
• Finally, go home, think about everything that you have seen and heard, and then make your decision.

CHANGING YOUR VET

If you move house, you may need to change your vet. In this case, you should select a new vet centre in the same way as before. When you register at the new centre, the receptionist there will contact your old centre to obtain your cat's medical records.

You may also wish to change your vet centre if you are unhappy with the service that you are receiving, but – before making a hasty decision – do talk through any grievance with an appropriate member of staff. It may well be that the problem has occurred because

To show you what to expect when you visit a vet centre, this is the interior plan of a typical centre with facilities to treat both dog and cat patients. On a tour of the centre you will be able to see behind the scenes, as well as the 'public' client areas.

of an unintentional breakdown in communications somewhere along the line, and it would be a pity to leave a good centre over a misunderstanding.

A SECOND OPINION

If your cat's condition does not seem to be improving despite treatment, your vet may suggest that he is seen by another vet. If this means taking your cat to another centre, your vet should make the arrangements.

At any time you may arrange a second opinion from another vet yourself, although some specialists

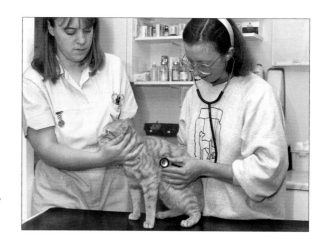

All vets are qualified to treat cats, but some will have a greater interest in them than others: bear this in mind when choosing the vet centre that will be best-suited to your cat's needs.

Health insurance

It is impossible to predict the cost of any veterinary care that your cat may need if he becomes ill. You can work out in advance the annual cost of preventive-healthcare procedures, but you cannot predict when he is going to be ill or when he may suffer an injury. And, if your cat does require veterinary treatment, there is no way of knowing how sophisticated that treatment will be, or for how long he will need it.

Veterinary fees are generally excellent value, when you consider the cost of the medical equipment used to treat cats, the cost of drugs and the advanced training of veterinary staff. However, unexpected bills from your vet centre can still make a dent in your cashflow.

Fortunately, it is now possible to insure against the cost of veterinary treatment, and many companies now offer a range of policies to suit the needs of cat-owners. For an annual premium, most policies will guarantee to pay all your veterinary fees up to a maximum amount in each year (you will probably have to pay an agreed sum towards each claim).

I would wholeheartedly recommend that you take out health insurance for your cat. I find nothing worse than seeing an owner, distraught about his or her cat's illness or injury, having to cope with the additional worry of how to pay for his care. You cannot expect your vet centre to reduce its fees because you do not have available funds: every vet centre is a business and must charge realistic fees to survive.

When choosing a health-insurance policy for your cat, be sure to read the small print. If in doubt, consult an insurance advisor. A typical policy may over broad cover, including the following:

• Veterinary fees for illness and accidents, including physiotherapy, hospitalization and referral.
• Cattery fees for your cat, or home-care with a friend, if you are taken into hospital for more than four days.
• Advertising and reward costs if your cat is lost.
• The cost of your cat will be reimbursed if he dies as the result of an accident or illness.

Unexpected veterinary fees can be an unwelcome burden. The chart below indicates the relative costs incurred in the first year of owning a pure-bred kitten who suffers a serious injury.

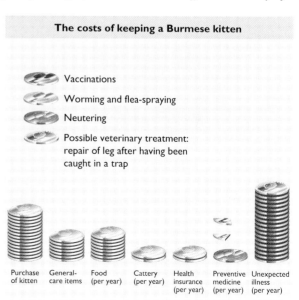

The costs of keeping a Burmese kitten

Vaccinations
Worming and flea-spraying
Neutering
Possible veterinary treatment: repair of leg after having been caught in a trap

Purchase of kitten | General-care items | Food (per year) | Cattery (per year) | Health insurance (per year) | Preventive medicine (per year) | Unexpected illness (per year)

Veterinary procedures

The best way to ensure that you and your cat get the most from the veterinary profession is to familiarize yourself with the services available from vet centres. With an understanding of some of the procedures that are commonly carried out, you will be able to make better-informed healthcare choices for your cat.

ACCIDENT-AND-EMERGENCY SERVICES

Very few vet centres are open 24 hours a day for their clients to turn up unannounced, but all centres (in the UK) have to provide accident-and-emergency services 24 hours a day, 365 days a year. If they cannot do so themselves, they will arrange access to the services of another vet centre in the same area.

Accident-and-emergency procedure

If you need veterinary help for your cat out of hours, you will normally have to telephone your vet centre. The telephone may be answered by a member of staff on duty, or by an answering machine. The machine will either give you another number to telephone, or will ask you to leave a message. It should automatically contact a vet or a nurse on duty, and you will be called back. One way or another, you will end up speaking directly to a vet or a veterinary nurse.

Remember that, out of hours, the vet or veterinary nurse to whom you speak may be unfamiliar to you. Equally, he or she may not know your cat personally, and may not have his records immediately available. Answer any questions accurately, and listen carefully to the instructions that you are given.

Your vet may wish to see your cat. A home visit may be essential in some cases, but if possible your vet will ask you to take your cat to the vet centre. With better facilities there than are available in the back of a car, it will be easier to examine and treat him.

Be sensible about how you use the out-of-hours services available from your vet centre. You should expect to pay a fee supplement for these services. (For further information on coping with accidents and emergencies, refer to pages 114–23.)

Your vet may use a number of pieces of diagnostic equipment to examine your cat, including an ophthalmoscope like this one to look in detail at his eyes.

CONSULTATIONS

During working hours, your vet centre should offer the option of an individual consultation with your vet, for him or her to examine your cat or to discuss any other health-related matter. Some centres also offer the option of a consultation with a veterinary nurse for minor procedures or healthcare advice.

'Open' surgeries are run on a first-come, first-seen basis, but many centres also offer appointments that may be booked in advance.

What is involved?

The length of a consultation will vary from centre to centre, but should take at least 15 minutes. In my view, it is not possible to examine a cat, question his owner, make a diagnosis and decide on a treatment in less time than this. Most centres organize surgeries several times a day, and some are open six or even seven days a week.

You should expect to be asked to pay a fixed fee for the appointment, plus an extra amount to cover the cost of any tests, drugs or other products that your vet uses.

DIAGNOSTICS

Diagnostic procedures are carried out in an attempt to identify the underlying cause or causes of symptoms that are shown by an ill cat. Many of these procedures – such as examinations using a stethoscope, an otoscope or an ophthalmoscope – will be carried out in your presence by your vet or a veterinary nurse in the consulting room.

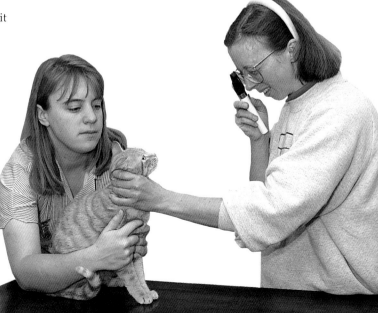

Carrying out tests

You should expect your cat to be admitted as an in-patient for procedures such as X-ray investigations, which may require the use of sophisticated equipment, or which can only be carried out with your cat sedated or anaesthetized (see pages 94–5). If your vet centre does not have the facilities needed to undertake certain diagnostic procedures, your vet will arrange for your cat to be examined elsewhere.

The procedures that are most commonly carried out on ill cats include the following:

Physical examination • A basic physical examination involves a systematic evaluation of a cat's external and internal anatomy, through observation and palpation. This procedure may include rectal or vaginal examination.

Temperature-taking • A cat's body temperature is recorded using a thermometer inserted into his rectum. Traditional mercury thermometers and electronic thermometers are both used. The rectal temperature of a normal cat is about 38.5°C (101.3°F).

Stethoscope examination • A stethoscope is a device that helps to amplify sounds within a cat's body, such as his heartbeat, the movements of air when he breathes, and the sounds created by the mixing and digestion of food in his stomach and intestines. Avoid talking to your vet when he or she is using a stethoscope, as you will make it difficult for him or her to hear some of the quieter sounds generated from within your cat's body. The heart-rate of a normal cat at rest is generally between 110 and 140 beats per minute; the breathing rate is usually between 24 and 42 breaths per minute.

Otoscope examination • An otoscope is an instrument used to examine a cat's ears. It has cone-shaped attachments designed to fit snugly into the ear holes, while a built-in light and magnifying lens provide a clear view of the dark depths of the ear canals. In a normal cat, the ear drum appears as a white sheet of tissue across the ear canal.

Ophthalmoscope examination • An ophthalmoscope is an instrument used to examine a cat's eyes. It has a built-in light, a number of filters and various lenses to allow examination of the anatomy of an eye in detail. The retina of a normal cat's eye makes a very colourful and beautiful image when viewed through an ophthalmoscope.

Endoscope examination • An endoscope is a special optical instrument that allows a vet to take a direct and detailed look at parts of a cat's anatomy that

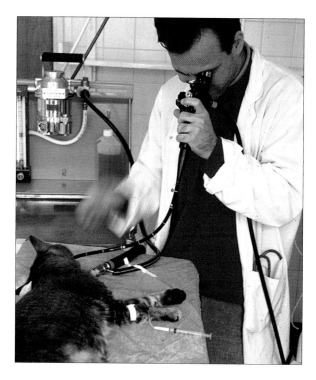

This vet is using an endoscope to look into the stomach of an anaesthetized cat. The controls on the eye-piece allow him to move the tip of the endoscope, in order to view different areas.

are normally hidden from view, such as deep inside his airways or down his oesophagus and into his stomach. Some endoscopes are rigid tubes; others are flexible pipes whose tips can be controlled. A cat will normally be anaesthetized during an endoscope examination (see pages 94–5).

X-ray investigation • The X-ray equipment in most vet centres is a smaller version of that used in human hospitals. The pictures created by an X-ray machine offer a view of a cat's internal anatomy. Bones are particularly easy to identify, as they appear white. Other structures are more difficult to visualize, and interpreting X-ray pictures takes experience. A cat is normally heavily sedated or anaesthetized during an X-ray investigation (see pages 94–5).

Ultrasound investigation • If you have had a baby, you will be very familiar with ultrasound machines. Not every vet centre has its own machine, but more and more are now obtaining them. These are highly sophisticated tools that create complex images of a cat's internal anatomy. Their most obvious and perhaps simplest use is in confirming pregnancy.

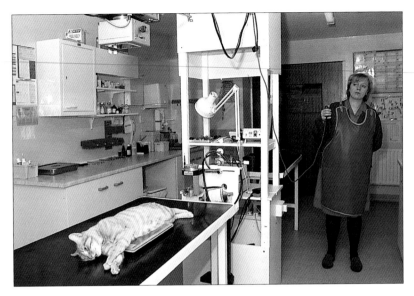

Almost all cats (with the exception of those who are critically ill) are sedated or anaesthetized for X-ray investigations. This is so that they remain still and a clear picture can be obtained.

Electrocardiography (ECG) examination • An ECG machine records electrical activity in a cat's beating heart, and is most often used to detect and identify abnormalities relating to the anatomy of the heart or the way in which it works. The procedure involves attaching a number of wires to the cat's skin, and is most often carried out with the cat lying on his side. In some cases, a cat may be fitted with a portable ECG unit that records the electrical activity in his heart over a prolonged period.

Laboratory procedures

It is likely that – at some point in his life – your cat will have samples taken from him for analysis. Some of the most common procedures are as follows:

Blood testing • Blood tests are carried out for many reasons, such as to assess a cat's body chemistry or the state of his immune system, or how well certain vital organs – including his liver and kidneys – are working. Samples of blood are taken either from the so-called cephalic vein in a foreleg, or from the larger jugular vein in the neck. The blood is then immediately stored in special containers before being analysed in a laboratory. Many vet centres have their own laboratories, but may send samples to outside laboratories for special tests; other centres will send away all their blood samples. A number of tests are

normally carried out on a blood sample at the same time; the results of this are called a blood profile.

Urine testing • Urine tests may be carried out for a number of reasons, including to check for abnormalities associated with urinary conditions, such as feline lower-urinary-tract disease (see pages 66–7), or to assess how well a cat's kidneys are working. Glucose is normally absent from a cat's urine, but will appear in the urine of a cat who is suffering from diabetes mellitus (see pages 70–1). You may be asked to obtain a urine sample from your cat. In this case, your vet or a nurse should provide you with a special litter-tray with washable litter, and will tell you how to use it.

Biopsy • This is a sample of a cat's tissue that is sent to a pathologist for examination of its microscopic structure. A biopsy will be taken under some form of anaesthesia (see pages 94–5), and is a common procedure for investigating unidentified growths.

Analysis of fluids • Your vet may send a sample of abnormal fluid – such as pus – to a laboratory to be cultured and examined. Any microscopic organisms that are associated with it can then be identifed.

TREATMENT PROCEDURES

Should he become ill, your cat may experience two types of conventional therapy: surgical treatments and medical treatments (or a combination of the two).

Surgical treatments

Dental descaling and polishing, neutering, midwifery, removing a broken claw, repairing a wound, mending a broken bone and removing a growth are just some of the many surgical procedures carried out at vet centres.

All vet centres, apart from the smallest clinic-only types, should have full surgical facilities. These will include all necessary general-anaesthetic equipment, an operating theatre stocked with surgical instruments and a post-anaesthetic recovery area. Some vet centres are also set up with specialist tools such as lasers and freezing equipment for cryosurgery (see page 50).

The facilities in some of the largest vet centres are very similar to those of human hospitals. Much of the surgical and anaesthetic equipment that they use will in fact have been developed for use on humans, and

SURGICAL FEES

Fees for any surgery carried out on your cat will consist of the cost of the anaesthetic, the operating-theatre time required and any other items used during the procedure, including cotton wool, syringes, needles and dressings.

Remember that the technical skills of the surgeon and the equipment required are very advanced, and that you must expect a fair but realistic bill.

then adapted for use on animals. It is now possible to carry out open-heart surgery on those cats who need it, but the complexity of the surgery that is undertaken at a particular vet centre will depend on its equipment and on the expertise of its staff.

Veterinary nurses may carry out minor surgical procedures – such as stitching a wound – on their own, and may assist vets with more major surgery such as repairing a ruptured diaphragm (see page 73). General anaesthetics are usually the responsibility of both a vet and a nurse (see pages 94–5).

Medical treatments

Medical treatments may be administered to cats using a variety of methods.

Drugs • These may be given in several ways, including by mouth or topically to the affected part of the body (see pages 101–3). Most of the medicines given to ill cats by vets and nurses are administered by injection. Injections may be given as follows:
- Under the skin, most commonly over the neck
- Into a muscle
- Directly into the bloodstream, most commonly via the cephalic vein in a foreleg.

Fluid therapy • This is the administration of special fluids into the bloodstream, and is a common and often life-saving procedure. A cat undergoing fluid therapy is often referred to as being 'on a drip'.

Blood transfusion • This may be carried out between cats when necessary.

DISPENSARY SERVICES

If your cat requires therapy using drugs, your vet or a veterinary nurse will normally begin his treatment at the vet centre, usually during a consultation. You will then be asked to continue administering the drugs to your cat at home.

Rather than supplying prescriptions, almost all vet centres (in the UK) run their own dispensary to supply drugs to their patients. This will generally be managed by a veterinary nurse, who will give you advice about how to use any drugs that your vet has prescribed for your cat (see also pages 101–3).

PSYCHIATRY SERVICES

Advice on coping with the simplest and most common behavioural problems of cats should be available from all good vet centres. Some centres employ individuals – often vets, nurses or zoologists – who have a special interest and expertise in helping owners to resolve more complex aspects of cat behaviour. A centre that does not offer such a service itself should be happy to refer clients to an animal-behaviour expert elsewhere.

SERVICES FOR HEALTHY CATS

Your vet centre is not just there for when things go wrong, but should also offer a range of other products and services that will help you to keep your cat healthy.

Your vet centre will almost certainly be able to vaccinate your cat (see page 85). A good centre should also supply a range of healthcare products, including those designed for dental care and parasite control, and may stock special commercially prepared diets to help in the treatment of specific conditions (see page 105).

Supplying you with products is only part of ensuring good healthcare for your cat – more important is the advice that you will need to select the most appropriate products and to use them properly. Your vet, or a nurse who is specially trained in all aspects of cat healthcare – including nutrition and cat behaviour – will give you invaluable advice. Veterinary nurses may offer advice either on a one-to-one basis or in group clinics.

REFERRALS

Very few vet centres have the equipment and expertise to provide clients with all the veterinary services that they may need. If your cat requires procedures that are not available at your centre, your vet may suggest that you take him to see another vet at another centre or at a special referral hospital.

If necessary, your vet should also be able to refer you to other professionals involved in animal care, such as animal-behaviour experts or even physiotherapists.

COMPLEMENTARY-THERAPY SERVICES

Complementary-therapy services are now becoming available to cat-owners through vet centres, and include homoeopathy, acupuncture and herbalism. If you would like your cat to be treated with complementary medicines whenever possible, make sure that your veterinary staff understand your wishes in advance.

Anaesthesia

Most cats will experience a general anaesthetic at some point in their lives, but the thought of their cats being anaesthetized and submitted to an operation is a cause of great concern to many owners, often due to fear of the unknown. The following outline of events that are likely to take place if your cat is admitted for an anaesthetic should help to put your mind at rest. (Note that the precise procedures will vary, depending on the reason for your cat's anaesthetic, and on the specific practices of the staff at your vet centre.)

The night before an anaesthetic

You will normally be asked to withhold all food from your cat after his dinner on the evening prior to the day of his anaesthetic. This is to make sure that he has an empty stomach when he is anaesthetized, as some of the drugs used may stimulate him to vomit. You should not need to restrict his access to water in any way.

Admission

You will normally be asked to bring your cat to the vet centre early in the morning on the day of his operation. You will be asked to sign a consent form, giving your authority for your cat to undergo specified procedures.

Examination and pre-medication

Your cat will be examined by your vet or a veterinary nurse to check that there is nothing unexpected wrong with him. You will be asked to confirm that he has not

Having had his 'pre-med', this cat is being given the first part of a general anaesthetic. The vet is injecting this into a tiny vein on the foreleg: the cat will be unconscious in seconds.

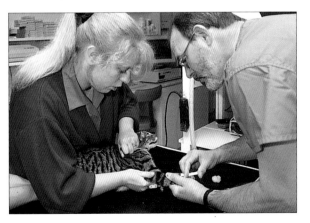

WHAT ARE ANAESTHETICS?

Anaesthetics allow a vet to carry out a diagnostic or surgical procedure safely and without causing pain. The following two anaesthetic procedures are used on cats:
• **Local analgesia:** drugs may be used as injections, sprays, creams or ointments to take away the sensation of pain from a part of the body. Surgical procedures carried out under local analgesia include removing small foreign bodies from the skin and treating minor wounds.
• **General anaesthesia:** anaesthetic drugs in the form of injectable liquids or breathable gases 'intoxicate' a cat's nervous system. They cause a loss of consciousness, prevent awareness of pain and relax the skeletal muscles.

eaten since the night before. Your vet or nurse will then give your cat one or more injections, often referred to as the 'pre-med'. This is likely to include a tranquillizer or sedative drug that will help to relieve any anxiety, and will also reduce the amount of general anaesthetic that is required later on.

You may feel reluctant to leave your cat, but he will adjust to the situation more quickly if you disappear without too much fuss. Although many vet centres are happy for owners to stay with their cats while the pre-med is administered, you may be encouraged to leave him before it is given.

The anaesthetic

As soon as the pre-med has taken effect and your vet is ready, your cat will be moved to a preparation room. Sitting or lying on a table, he will have a small area of fur clipped from one foreleg, close to his elbow. This will be the place where the first part of the anaesthetic will be injected into his cephalic vein.

Within seconds of the liquid anaesthetic entering the vein, your cat's legs will start to weaken and he will be helped to a lying position on his side. He will already be completely unconscious.

Your vet will then pass a breathing pipe called an endotracheal tube down into your cat's windpipe, and the end of the tube will be connected to an anaesthetic machine. From this point onwards, your cat will be breathing a mixture of one or more anaesthetic gases and oxygen. The veterinary nurse will monitor his respiration, pulse rate and degree of unconsciousness, and will adapt the anaesthetic as necessary.

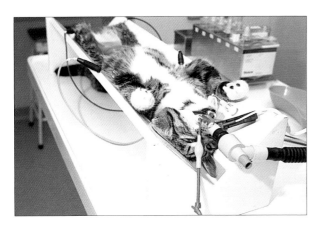

With modern equipment and advanced anaesthetic techniques, vets are able to carry out major surgical procedures that would not have been attempted in the past. This anaesthetized cat will be covered with sterile drapes before his operation begins.

Preparation

If your cat is to undergo surgery, the area of his body in which an incision is to be made will be clipped, and the skin will be cleaned with antibacterial solution. He will then be moved to the operating theatre, where the cleaning process will be repeated.

Meanwhile, your vet and any assistants will prepare themselves by scrubbing their hands with antibacterial soap and putting on sterile gowns, hats and gloves. Your vet will cover your cat's body – except the area where the incision will be made – with sterile drapes.

The operation or procedure

Your vet will carry out the operation or procedure as quickly as is safe and feasible, so that your cat remains anaesthetized for the shortest time possible.

Recovery

The level of the anaesthetic will be reduced when your vet is close to finishing the surgery. Your cat will be disconnected from the anaesthetic machine and taken to a recovery ward where he will be kept comfortable while he wakes up. A nurse may administer further drugs – such as painkillers – and will monitor him.

The speed with which your cat wakes up will depend on his age, general state of health and the anaesthetic drugs used. If he is young and healthy and has undergone a routine procedure, he will probably regain consciousness in minutes and may be sitting up within half an hour. A nurse will continue to monitor his recovery.

Discharge from the vet centre

Most cats who are anaesthetized for routine procedures go home the same day. When you collect your cat, your vet or a veterinary nurse will give you specific advice regarding his home nursing, and will tell you when they would like to see him again.

Your cat should be able to walk, although he may still be a little drowsy. You may be surprised at how bright and bouncy he is, but this does not mean that you should treat him just as normal: after a general anaesthetic, he will need special and appropriate nursing care (see below and pages 98–111).

At home

When you get home, take your cat to his bed and encourage him to rest. Use a wrapped hot-water bottle or other heat source (see page 106) to keep him warm. Make sure that his cat flap is closed, and that he cannot venture outdoors. Confine him to one room, or to a cage if appropriate (see page 106), and provide one or more litter-trays. Unless you have been advised otherwise, offer your cat a small meal if he is interested in food. Ensure that water is nearby for him to drink if he is thirsty. Then leave him to rest, but keep an eye on him.

Keep your cat calm and quiet for the next few days, and strictly follow the advice that you have been given about his exercise and general management.

Before any procedure is carried out on your cat, make sure that you understand fully what will be done, and why. If he is to undergo surgery, you will be asked to sign a consent form.

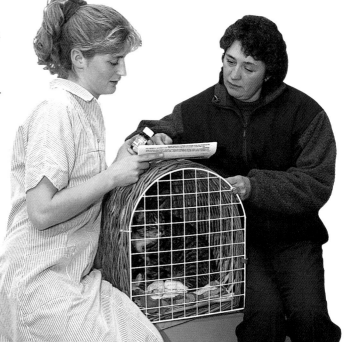

Products used in treatment

There is a very wide range of drugs, preparations and other products available to help treat, control or prevent diseases and conditions that affect cats. These include the following:

• Conventional medicines, such as antibiotics and anti-inflammatory drugs (see below and opposite).

• Special drug preparations including creams and ointments for topical use.

• Special fluids, which may be given to a cat who is either unwilling or unable to take in sufficient fluids by mouth in order to prevent him from becoming dehydrated. These are administered intravenously, via a 'drip' (see page 93).

• Vaccines, which are used to protect cats from the major infectious diseases (see pages 80–5). Your vet or a veterinary nurse will advise you on the vaccinations that your cat requires (see also page 113); these will need to be administered at your vet centre.

• Products suitable for preventing infestations of the common parasites of cats (see pages 28–9 and 54–8) may be available from a number of different sources, but your vet centre is likely to stock a comprehensive range of the most up-to-date products.

• Prepared 'prescription' diets are specially formulated foods that are designed to help in the treatment of a range of diseases and conditions (see page 105).

• Complementary medicines, such as homoeopathic and herbal remedies (see page 93).

Giving medicines at home

When your cat is unwell and needs medical treatment, your vet will create a specific treatment regime for him. This regime may contain just one kind of medicine, or may involve a combination of drugs, preparations and other products.

It is likely that your cat's initial treatment will be carried out by your vet or a veterinary nurse; you will then be supplied with all that you need to continue the treatment regime at home. You should be given precise instructions as to the size and timing of any drug doses, and these details should also be printed clearly on the labels of the medicine containers.

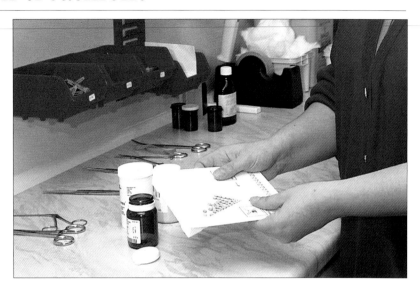

On the instructions of your vet, a nurse will normally prepare the medicines and any other products selected as part of your cat's treatment, while you wait. Everything should be clearly labelled, with detailed dosage and administration information.

Perhaps the most common drugs prescribed for the treatment of cats are antibiotics and anti-inflammatory drugs. However, in my experience few owners – even those who have been prescribed such drugs themselves by a doctor – actually know much about them.

ANTIBIOTICS

Antibiotics are drugs that are used to help in the control of bacterial infections. They either kill the bacteria that are sensitive to their effects, or prevent those bacteria from reproducing. 'Specific' antibiotics are most effective at controlling infections by certain types of bacteria, while so-called 'broad-spectrum' antibiotics are effective against the widest range of bacteria.

Antibiotics may be administered in the form of tablets, capsules, powders or injections, and may be included in ointments, creams and other preparations for external (topical) use (see pages 101–3).

You should be aware that, if antibiotics are not used appropriately, bacteria may develop resistance to their actions. As a result, if antibiotics are prescribed for your cat, it is very important that you do not miss any doses. It is also essential that you complete the full course of treatment, even if your cat appears to have recovered.

ANTI-INFLAMMATORY DRUGS

These types of drugs are prescribed for a variety of conditions, and fall into the following major categories.

Corticosteroids

These drugs are often simply referred to as 'steroids'. They are very powerful drugs that have marked and wide-ranging effects within a cat's body, even when they are only administered in very small doses. They are generally used to control severe inflammation.

Steroids cause a number of well known side-effects. These invlude mood changes and increased thirst as a result of the production of larger-than-normal volumes of urine by treated individuals. Because of their many side-effects, corticosteroids should only be used in the lowest effective doses for the shortest possible time. Treatment with these drugs is normally withdrawn gradually at the end of a course.

Corticosteroids may be administered as tablets or by injection, and may be included in creams, ointments, drops and other preparations for external (topical) use.

Non-steroidal anti-inflammatory drugs

These drugs are most commonly used to lower the body temperature of a cat with fever, and as painkillers. Cats are particularly susceptible to being poisoned by

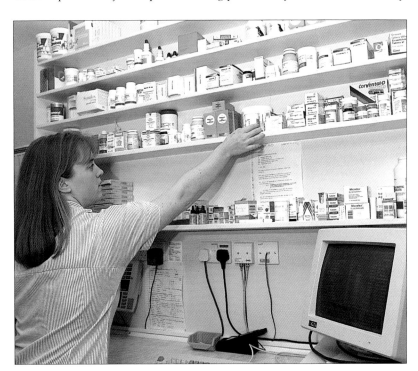

these kinds of drugs, so never administer any of your own anti-inflammatory drugs (aspirin is an example) to your cat without first consulting your vet.

AVAILABILITY OF MEDICINES

The availability of medicines is strictly controlled by law. For example, in the UK all drugs intended for use on cats currently have to be licensed by a government body called the Veterinary Medicines Directorate.

In general, the most powerful drugs – as well as some newly developed medicines – are only available to cat-owners from vet centres at which the owners are registered as clients.

Certain less-powerful drugs, with well-established safety records, may also be sold by pharmacies to members of the general public. The drugs that are considered safest of all by the Veterinary Medicines Directorate may be available over the counter in any appropriate retail shop.

STORING MEDICINES

If tablets or capsules are prescribed for your cat, they should be given to you in 'child-proof' containers. However, you must still ensure that all medicines are stored in a secure place where they are well out of the reach of children, and where your cat cannot get to them.

You should regularly check the 'use-by' dates on medicines in your medicine cabinet. If you find any that are out of date, wrap them up and then dispose of them safely (perhaps the best way is to take them back to your vet centre).

Most vet centres have their own drugs dispensary that will carry a stock of a very wide range of drugs. If your cat is on permanent medication of any kind, make sure that you always obtain new supplies before he actually needs them.

Special care

There are times in your cat's life when he will require very special care, such as when he is ill or recovering from an operation, or when he is simply growing old. For however long it is necessary, your cat's care will become one of your main priorities: he will need your time, as well as your love and concern.

Handling and restraining your cat

The type of care that your cat is likely to need if he is ill or injured will depend on his condition, and on the procedure that he has undergone at your vet centre.

Your vet or a veterinary nurse will tell you exactly what needs doing and how to do it, and, the closer the contact you keep with your vet centre, the easier you will find it to care for your cat.

Your responsibilities may include carrying out any or all of the following tasks:
• Administering any medicines prescribed by your vet (see pages 101–3).
• Attending to any special dietary needs that your cat may have (see pages 104–5).
• Attending to your cat's comfort and personal-hygiene needs (see page 107).
• Adjusting his lifestyle as necessary (see page 107).
• Attending to the care of any wounds and dressings (see pages 108–9).
• Monitoring your cat's condition, and reporting back to your vet centre (see pages 110–11).

If, for whatever reason, you are unwilling or unable to carry out any of the specific nursing tasks that you are asked to perform, you must tell your vet, who will do all that he or she can to help you make alternative arrangements for your cat's care.

HANDLING YOUR CAT
When carrying out any examination or procedure on your cat, it is essential that you know how to handle him appropriately. Your cat may not appreciate what you have to do to him, but a well-practised and slick approach will ensure that any discomfort on his part is felt for as brief a time as possible.

By adopting the correct technique, you should be able to carry out any nursing task both quickly and

effectively, without putting your safety at risk. Proper restraint is even more important when your cat is ill or injured, as his behaviour may become unpredictable if he is in pain. If possible, you should always have an assistant. One of you can then restrain your cat, while the other carries out the procedure.

RESTRAINT TECHNIQUES
You should avoid trying to restrain your cat on the ground, unless his condition makes it inappropriate to lift him. An old table with a non-slip surface makes an ideal examination and treatment bench.

Always try to match the degree of restraint to the procedure that you wish to carry out: the general rule of animal nursing is to use the minimum restraint that is necessary to ensure control. Be firm but kind, and be sensitive to your cat's mood. If you are not sufficiently firm, your cat may sense this and try to escape; if you are too firm, he may panic. Talk to him, as he will find your voice reassuring, and try to make the experience of being handled for an unusual and a potentially uncomfortable procedure – such as the administration of ear drops – as pleasant for him as possible.

Remember that you may well need to administer a course of medication, and that the next dose may only be a few hours away. Confine your cat indoors when he is on medication, as, having been treated once, he may be less than keen to return home for a re-run.

If you have difficulties
Despite your best efforts, your cat may become very upset when you try to restrain him to carry out a physical examination or procedure. If this is the case, do not persevere. Once agitated, few cats calm down but instead become more and more frantic. If you were

Restraining your cat in a lying position

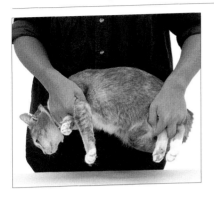

1 With your cat on a suitable table, lean over him and grasp the foreleg and hindleg nearest to you. Slowly but firmly, lift these legs off the table and away from your body: your cat will slide down your front.

2 Adjust your hold to rest the arm restraining your cat's forelegs over his neck, and move your other arm over his bottom. Hold him gently but firmly in this position.

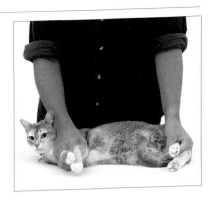

attempting to restrain your cat on your own, leave him for a while (keeping him indoors) and then try again later when you can ask someone else to help you. If no one is available to assist you, contact your vet centre: your vet or a veterinary nurse will advise you as to what action to take, and may well suggest that you put your cat in his carrying basket and take him to the vet centre so that he or she can help you.

You should regularly practise basic handling techniques on your cat. In this way, you will quickly become an accomplished handler and he should become a resigned and patient patient! You should start this as soon as you bring your cat home as a young kitten. The best time to practise will be during his routine weekly health-checks (see pages 8–9).

The following are some of the most important basic restraint techniques.

Picking up your cat

Pick up your cat by placing both hands around his chest. Then, as you lift him, tuck his rear end in against your body, under your elbow. Adjust the hand position of that arm so that it supports his chest, and hold on to his forelegs with the fingers of that hand.

Your other hand will now be free: use this to stroke your cat's neck gently, as this will help to make him feel more relaxed. If he tries to jump free, you will also be able to grasp him quickly by his scruff (see below).

Emergency confinement

If your cat suddenly becomes ill or is injured, it may be impossible to handle him because he is so frightened and/or aggressive. In this case, try to get him into his carrying basket straight away as, once he is confined, he will not be able to escape. You can then take him quickly and safely to your vet centre, where the staff will take care of him (see also page 117).

'Scruffing'

When handling your cat, one of your main priorities is to prevent his claws and teeth from coming into contact with your skin. If he is extremely well-behaved you may only need to support his head in a cupped hand, but if he moves quickly as a result of pain, such a technique may not be adequate.

A much better way to gain control over your cat's head is to grasp as much spare skin as you can over his neck,

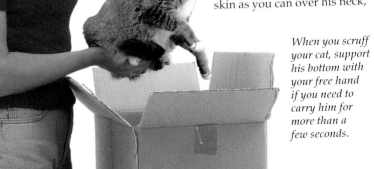

When you scruff your cat, support his bottom with your free hand if you need to carry him for more than a few seconds.

and to hold on to this skin tightly. This technique is known as 'scruffing'. When he is 'scruffed', your cat may become resigned to his fate without you having to hold on to his skin very tightly, so be sure to adjust the strength of your grip in response to his behaviour.

From the expression on your cat's face you may well imagine that by scruffing him you are hurting him, but this is very unlikely unless you are being excessively heavy-handed. His expression will probably be the result of you pulling the skin taut over his face.

Scruffing is also the technique that you should use if you need to seize your cat in an emergency (see also page 116), or to retrieve him from a hiding place such as behind the washing machine or up a tree!

HANDLING EQUIPMENT

Special handling bags are a high-tech way of achieving the same result as towelling (see below). These bags are designed for a cat to be zipped up inside, with just his head peeping out. Zipped openings in the corners then provide access to different parts of the body. These bags are a very good idea, especially for owners who may not have assistants available when handling their cats.

Muzzles – which are actually more like face-masks – are also available for cats. These are made of nylon fabric, and are designed to subdue and calm a cat

during a handling procedure, on the principle that what a cat cannot see will not worry him. This is a good idea in theory, but is often less successful in practice.

SAFETY FIRST

Just because your cat is normally very docile, do not make the mistake of assuming that he will be equally calm when he is ill, in pain or on the receiving end of a particularly foul-tasting tablet.

Never put yourself at risk when giving medicines to your cat, or when he is in pain (see also pages 114–16). Cat scratches and bites are not only painful but can also make you seriously ill, and it is always best to be over-cautious. If you are scratched or bitten by your cat, you should contact your doctor (see page 60).

'Towelling'

In my experience, if a person tries to carry out even a simple procedure on a cat's head without the help of an assistant, the cat suddenly seems to develop legs everywhere. He will rapidly become impossible to keep still, and may well use his claws in an attempt to avoid being treated.

If you have to administer medicine by mouth to your cat, or if you need to treat any part of his head such as his eyes or ears, and you do not have anyone available to help you to restrain him properly, wrap him tightly in a large towel.

The standard wrapping procedure can be adapted to leave one leg – as well as the cat's head – out of the towel. If you would like a demonstration of the technique, ask your vet or a nurse to show you.

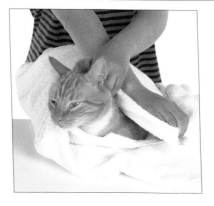

1 Lay a large towel out flat. Scruff your cat, and place him along the centre of the towel. Without letting go of his scruff, use your other hand to wrap one side of the towel tightly over your cat's back. Tuck it just under his body on the other side.

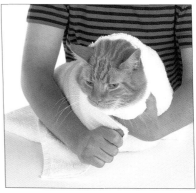

2 Wrap the rest of the towel over your cat in the other direction, and only then let go of his scruff to finish wrapping the towel beneath his body. (If your cat pokes his front feet through the neck hole, you will need to wrap him more tightly.)

Administering medicines

Most ill cats will be treated as out-patients of vet centres, and your vet or nurse may ask you to administer medicines to your cat at home when he is unwell. In addition, even when your cat is healthy you will need to medicate him regularly to prevent well-known common conditions such as parasitic-worm infestations (see pages 28–9).

Always read very carefully the instructions on any type of medication, and follow strictly any additional recommendations offered by your vet or a veterinary nurse. He or she should be happy to give a practical demonstration, if you are unsure about a particular administration technique.

If you do not feel confident about administering a medicine at home to your cat, make sure that you tell your vet. He or she may be able to prescribe a treatment designed to be administered in a different way, or may be willing to arrange for your cat to have his medication administered at your vet centre as and when necessary. Never pretend that you have administered medication to your cat when you have not done so.

Safety first

Few cats are easy-going enough to tolerate being medicated without some fuss, so always try to arrange for someone else to help you. Another pair of hands will make the task less stressful for both you and your cat, and you are more likely to administer any medicine successfully at the first attempt. If you cannot summon assistance, wrap your cat in a towel (see opposite).

Avoid medicating your cat on the ground or on your lap. You are much more likely to be able to keep control over him if he is on unfamiliar territory, such as a table-top. Make sure that this has a non-slip surface.

Giving liquids and syrups

Before you start, check the dose on the medicine container, and shake a liquid if this is specified. Ask your assistant to restrain your cat from behind, and to hold on tightly to his forelegs.

Draw up the correct dose of medicine into the supplied dropper or syringe. Support your cat's head firmly with one hand and place the end of the dropper or syringe into the side of his mouth, just behind his canine tooth. Aiming across his mouth – not towards his throat – gently administer the liquid or syrup.

Your cat may try to chew at the dropper or syringe as the medicine goes into his mouth, but this will actually encourage him to swallow it. If at any point he starts to cough, immediately lower his head. Wait for him to settle down, then try again more slowly.

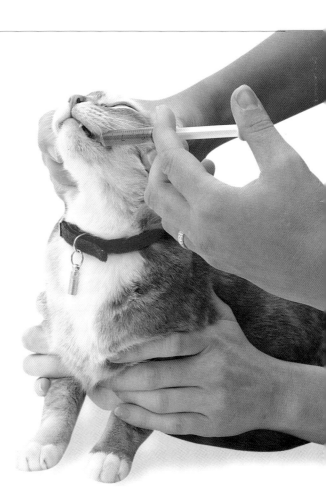

MEDICINES IN FOOD

Some – but not all – medicines may be mixed into food to make their administration easier. Cats are very good at detecting 'doctored' food, so choose a very smelly moist food that your cat finds palatable, and pre-heat it to body temperature before mixing in the medicine. This will help to release pleasant odours from the food and should help to disguise the smell of the medication.

Giving tablets and capsules

Tablets and capsules are normally given by mouth. Understandably, cats resent being force-fed with medicines in any form, and few will take them in this way voluntarily.

Before you begin, check the dose on the medicine container. Ask an assistant to hold your cat's forelegs to restrain him in a sitting position.

1 Place the palm of your hand on your cat's head so that the edge of your index finger is just above his eyes, then curve your thumb and index finger around his eyes to press firmly on the bones beneath his lower eyelids. Gently turn your cat's face towards the ceiling until his lower jaw starts to open.

USEFUL TIPS

• Tablets with a dry, powdery surface may slip down more easily if you coat them in a little butter or margarine.
• Large tablets will be easier to give if you break them into smaller pieces, but do not do so without checking on the instructions or asking your vet, as some medicines may lose their effectiveness if tampered with.

• If you are worried about using your fingers, you could try a 'pill-popper'. This is just like a syringe: the tablet fits into a clasp at one end, and when you push the plunger the tablet is forced out. (Note: some pill-poppers advise part-filling with water, but I would advise against this as you could spray water into your cat's windpipe.)

2 With the tablet held between the index finger and thumb of your free hand, use your middle finger to open your cat's mouth. Drop in the tablet or capsule so that it falls on to the back of his tongue.

3 Quickly close your cat's mouth, and keep him looking skywards by supporting his head under his chin. Gently rub down his throat with your fingers to encourage him to swallow.

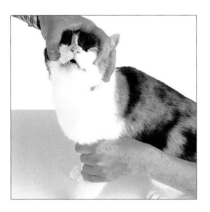
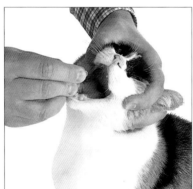
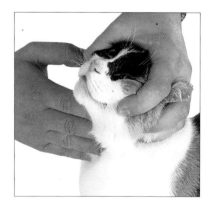

Administering eye drops

Gently wipe away any discharge from around your cat's eye or eyes using cotton wool dampened with plain water, or special eye-wipes. Check the medicine dose, and shake the drops if necessary.

Ask a helper to hold on to your cat's forelegs so that he is properly restrained. Take the bottle between the thumb and index finger of one hand, and support your cat's head

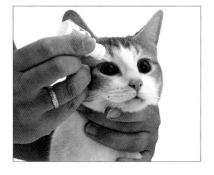

with the other. If he keeps his eyes closed, move the hand that is under his chin so that you can use the thumb of that hand to hold back the skin above his eye.

Squeeze the required number of drops on to your cat's eyeball, then release his head and allow him to blink several times: this will help to disperse the medicine over the surface of his eyeball.

Administering eye ointment

Carefully wipe away any discharge from your cat's eye or eyes using cotton wool wetted with water, or special eye-wipes. Check the dose on the medicine label.

With your cat properly restrained, hold on to his head with one hand and gently pull back on the skin above his upper eyelid using a finger or thumb. Hold the tube of ointment parallel to his eyelid, and then very carefully squeeze out the required amount so that it falls on to the edge of your cat's lower eyelid.

Release your cat's head and allow him to blink once or twice. Finally, carefully massage his upper and lower eyelids (while they are closed) to smear the ointment over the surface of the eyeball.

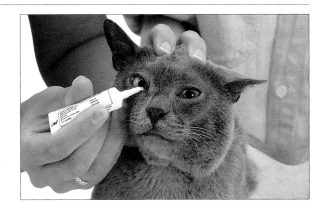

Administering ear drops or ointment

Check the dose on the medicine label, and shake the ear drops if necessary. Gently but thoroughly clean away any discharge that has accumulated around your cat's ear hole and on the inner side of his ear flap, using cotton wool wetted with plain water or with a proper ear-cleaning solution recommended by your vet centre.

When administering ear drops or ointment to your cat, it may be difficult for you to see exactly how much you are giving. For this reason, it may be a good idea to practise first into a sink to see how hard you have to squeeze the tube or bottle in order to deliver the correct amount of medicine.

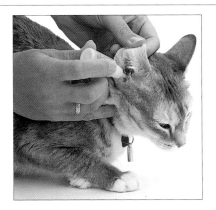

1 Hold your cat's ear flap between the thumb and first finger of one hand, and hold the nozzle of the medicine container just above his ear hole. Administer the medicine.

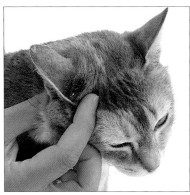

2 Your cat may shake his head, but hold on to his ear and massage the base of it to encourage the drops or ointment to flow down to his ear drum, past the bend in his ear canal.

FURTHER TIPS ON GIVING MEDICINES

KEEP YOUR CAT INDOORS
Even if your cat does not seem to be very ill, make sure that you keep him inside whenever he is on a course of medication. By doing so, you will be able to monitor his recovery, and you will know where to find him when he is due for a dose of medicine.

FINISH THE COURSE
Always complete the administration of a course of medication prescribed for your cat. Do not stop treatment because you think that his symptoms have improved, as many medicine courses are designed to be continued for a few days after apparent recovery.

If you cease treatment too early, your cat's illness may recur.

CONTACT YOUR VET CENTRE
If you have any problems in medicating your cat, or if he appears to have any reaction to being medicated, contact your vet centre immediately.

Food and drink

If specific dietary manipulations are appropriate to your cat's case management, your vet or veterinary nurse will advise you accordingly. It is likely that he or she will suggest basing your cat's diet while he is ill on a commercially prepared 'prescription' food formulated to help in the treatment or control of his condition.

SPECIAL NUTRITIONAL NEEDS

Dietary adjustments feature prominently in the treatment regimes for a number of major conditions. The following are just some examples:

• A cat suffering from diarrhoea (see pages 32–3) will benefit from highly digestible, low-fat meals fed on a little-and-often basis.

• A cat who has chronic renal failure (see pages 64–5) may benefit from a diet that is restricted in protein, phosphorus and sodium.

• A cat with struvite urolithiasis (see pages 66–7) may be treated by feeding a diet that has a direct effect on his urine and helps to dissolve the uroliths.

• An obese cat needs precisely controlled calorie restriction (see pages 76–7).

Although complete anorexia (refusal to eat) in a cat can lead to a life-threatening liver condition called hepatic lipidosis (see page 74), a short period of eating less than normal in a healthy cat is not thought to cause serious problems because his body has in-built mechanisms to compensate for the temporary lack of nutrition.

However, a cat whose body is stressed by disease, injury or surgery may suffer from much more serious

WARNING

Do not attempt to force-feed your cat without first consulting your vet. To prevent him from accidentally inhaling the liquid food – a situation that may lead to very serious consequences – you must make sure that your cat's head is not tipped far back, and that you give no more than 1–2 ml (¼ teaspoonful) of food or liquid at a time. Wait for your cat to swallow between doses.

symptoms as a result of even short periods of under-nourishment. The precise problems to which such a cat may be prone will depend on the kind of stress and its degree and severity, but may include the following:

• A decrease in his liver and muscle energy stores, forcing him to burn off his own tissues to provide his body processes with fuel. From a few days after being stressed by serious illness, injury or surgery, and for the following days or weeks, he may burn up more energy than normal. For example, after minor surgery he may use 10 per cent more fuel; if he suffers from a severe burn, his energy requirement may increase much more.

• Adverse effects on the immune system, leading to increased susceptibility to infections.

• Muscle wastage

• Abnormalities in the digestive system, making it more difficult for the cat to digest food.

• Shock

• Delayed wound healing

Administering solid food using a syringe

1 Ask your vet for a suitable-sized syringe, and cut off the end. Pull out the plunger and then push the cut-off syringe into the food so that you scoop a core of food into it.

2 Hold the syringe close to your cat's nose so that he can smell the food. As he opens his mouth, insert the syringe and gently push the plunger to deliver the food on to his tongue. If your cat will not open his mouth voluntarily, you may need to do this (see page 102).

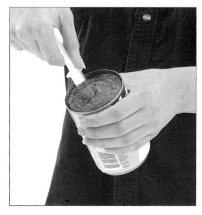
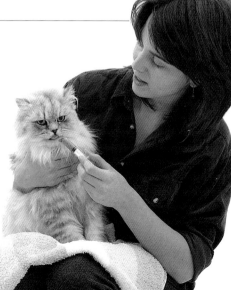

Avoiding under-nourishment

If your cat has not eaten normal amounts of food for three to five days as a result of illness, injury or surgery, or if he is suffering from significant muscle wastage as a result of illness, your vet may wish to incorporate the following in his diet:

• Fat as the main source of energy
• Sufficient protein to support normal growth
• Sufficient amounts of vitamins, minerals and essential fatty acids to support normal growth.
• Increased amounts of zinc

Special diets

There are now numerous prepared foods available that have been formulated to help in the treatment of certain conditions. These include foods to meet the special dietary needs of 'stressed' cats who do not wish to eat. They come in a highly palatable, liquid form that can be administered by syringe if necessary (see opposite, below) and are high in calories, so only small volumes are required to supply an ill cat's nutritional needs.

Your vet should give you very specific advice on how much to feed. The daily food allocation is normally best split between five or six small meals.

FEEDING AN ILL CAT

Ensuring that an ill cat receives adequate nourishment takes time, patience and often ingenuity. The following are some of the techniques commonly employed:
• Warming up the food to body temperature – about 38.5°C (101.3°F) – to release its odour.
• Removing any uneaten food after about 15 minutes: fresh food offered later will be more acceptable.
• Smearing small amounts of food on the lips
• Liquidizing the food
• Feeding the cat by hand

Forced feeding

A cat who will not eat voluntarily must be force-fed. The most common methods include the following:
• Placing small lumps of food on the back of the cat's tongue and encouraging him to swallow. The technique is similar to that used to give tablets and capsules by mouth (see pages 101–2) although, rather than placing the food by hand in your cat's mouth, you will find it easier to use a cut-off syringe (see opposite).
• Administering liquid food by mouth using a syringe. However, forced feeding may cause a cat undue stress. In this case, he may be fitted with a feeding tube to deliver liquid food directly into his digestive system.

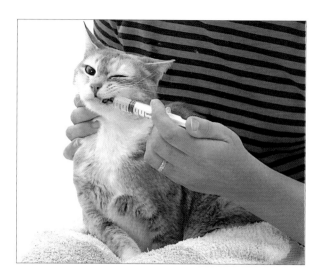

To give fluids to your cat, place the syringe tip between his side teeth. Aiming across his mouth, gently push the plunger.

FLUIDS

A cat can survive for weeks without food, but will remain alive for just a few days at the most without water. A typical cat contains over 2 litres (3½ pints) of water, accounting for 60 per cent of his body weight. He will constantly lose water in his faeces and urine, in the air he breathes out, in the sweat he produces through his feet and nose, and in other body secretions.

Water for a healthy cat

An average adult cat requires a minimum of about 200 ml (⅓ pint) of water per day. Some will be produced as his body burns up food, but most will come as part of his food or through drinking. Always give your cat access to water so that he can drink when he wishes.

Water for an ill cat

When your cat is recovering from illness, you should monitor how much he drinks (see page 110). Your vet will advise you if you need to give him extra water to prevent dehydration: the technique is similar to that for giving liquid medicines (see page 101).

Special fluids

Your vet may advise that you give your cat a special fluid to drink, to replace important chemicals that he may have lost as a result of vomiting or diarrhoea. Prepared powders are available, or you can make up a solution of 5 ml (1 teaspoonful) salt and 10 ml (one dessertspoonful) glucose to 2 litres (3½ pints) water.

Environment and personal hygiene

Offering your cat a quiet, peaceful and warm place to rest will help his convalescence after illness or injury. Your vet or a veterinary nurse should give you specific advice relating to your cat's basic management during this period: his or her precise recommendations will depend on the nature and severity of the condition.

For instance, recovery from routine surgery should be very straightforward, and your main management priority may lie in controlling your cat's general activity by simply keeping him confined in your house until his stitches are taken out. However, if your cat has been seriously ill or has undergone a major surgical procedure, his management when he returns home is likely to be much more complex, and may involve you caring for his personal-hygiene requirements and even taking on the role of his physiotherapist.

The following are some of the management issues relating to the nursing care of a convalescing cat.

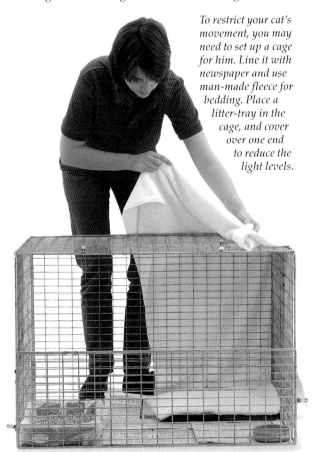

To restrict your cat's movement, you may need to set up a cage for him. Line it with newspaper and use man-made fleece for bedding. Place a litter-tray in the cage, and cover over one end to reduce the light levels.

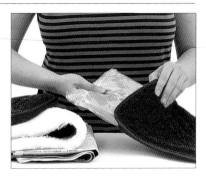

To keep your cat warm, you can place wrapped hot-water bottles near him (never put these directly against his skin). An alternative is to use special heat-generating packs: these are now widely available.

Your cat's bed

This should be in an out-of-the-way place, but where you can easily keep an eye on him. If he is weak or otherwise disabled, the bed must be close to the floor but away from any drafts. His environment should be quiet and warm, with low light levels.

Confinement

Your vet may advise that your cat is 'cage-rested': this means that his activity must be restricted to lying down, sitting, standing and turning around. The easiest way to achieve this is to use a wire-framed crate of the appropriate size; an alternative is to fence off a suitable area of a room with boarding or similar material.

No matter how confined your cat must be, he should still be able to move around enough to find a position that is comfortable for him to lie in. Only he knows which parts of him hurt the most!

Some hyperactive cats require short-term sedation during their convalescence, in order to make them rest.

Special bedding

Your cat's bedding should be warm, soft and easy to wash. The bedding used in most vet centres is a type of man-made fleece: this can be washed in a conventional washing machine and dries very quickly.

Warmth

You can keep your cat warm in a number of ways, without making his environment stuffy.
• You can place a hot water bottle in his bed (this must be covered and not placed in direct contact with your cat's skin).
• Electric heated pads are a good alternative, and are designed to be placed under a cat's bedding.
• Place blankets over him.

Toileting

Make sure that your cat has access at all times to a clean litter-tray, containing litter to which he is accustomed. If he does not normally use a litter-tray, you should offer him more than one tray, containing different kinds of litter (one of these should contain garden soil).

Position the litter-tray or trays as far away as you can from your cat's food and water. If he is confined to a cage, put the tray and his water bowl in opposite corners, and remove the tray when you feed him.

If your cat is unable to move, he will be forced to urinate and defecate where he lies. Incontinence may also be directly associated with his condition. Your cat may be upset about soiling his bed, so it is important that you clean up after him regularly. Old towels or babies' nappies opened up and placed underneath his bedding will soak up urine and help to keep him dry.

Hair care

If your cat has long hair, you must keep it clean and well-groomed. If it remains soiled or becomes matted, your cat may suffer from skin problems that will make him uncomfortable and may complicate his condition.

If he is incontinent, it may be sensible to trim away any long hair from under his tail and down the backs of his legs. Smearing petroleum jelly around his genitals and anus will help to prevent urine-scalding of the skin. Despite your efforts to prevent your cat from soiling his coat, you may still need to bathe him regularly.

For cats who enjoy it, grooming may also have a therapeutic effect (see also page 51).

Claw care

If your cat needs to be confined for a long period, and therefore cannot exercise normally, his claws may well become overgrown. Ask your vet or a veterinary nurse to cut them for him when he has a routine check-up, or very carefully trim them yourself. Provided that you have a sharp pair of clippers designed for cats' claws, the technique is straightforward (see page 63).

Personal hygiene

If your cat's mouth is dry, moisten it for him by wiping his gums with a damp sponge, gently squeezing out a little water as you wipe. You must make sure that he is fully awake when you do this, so that he can swallow any excess water.

Regularly wipe away any discharges that may accumulate at your cat's nose, eyes or at the corners of his mouth, using moist face-wipes.

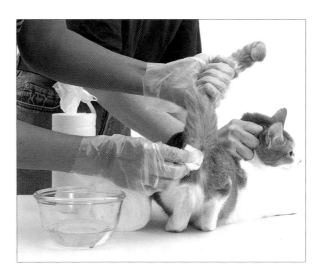

When your cat is ill, he may soil the area under his tail. To keep his bottom as clean and hygienic as possible, wash away the worst of any soiling using warm water and cotton wool, then gently finish cleaning the area using wet-wipes.

Mental and physical stimulation

Your cat will welcome the reassurance of your touch and the familiar sound of your voice, so spend time simply stroking and talking to him.

As you stroke him, try gently massaging your cat's skin and muscles to stimulate the circulation. You should avoid letting him lie in one position for too long: if he cannot move himself, turn him every few hours.

Physiotherapy

By gently manipulating your cat's joints, you will help to prevent stiffness. Your vet may ask you to carry out specific physiotherapy techniques to aid recovery.

Exercise

Follow the advice offered by your vet regarding the exercise that your cat should take. This may involve keeping him indoors until he has fully recovered and has finished any course of medication.

WARNING

If your cat is convalescing and on a course of medication, you should not allow him to go outdoors, even if he is not disabled in any way. This is so that you can carefully monitor his recovery (see pages 110–11) and administer any necessary treatments at the correct times.

Wound management

If your cat is recovering from a traumatic or a surgical wound, or from an uncomfortable skin condition, it is important that he does not damage the affected area further or interfere with the normal healing process through continued licking, biting or scratching as he attempts to relieve any irritation that he feels.

PROTECTING A WOUND

The method that will be used to help prevent this type of self-trauma will depend on the nature of your cat's wound or skin condition, the degree of irritation that it is causing, the part of the body affected, your cat's temperament and your availability to supervise him.

An 'Elizabethan collar' is a simple device to prevent a cat from scratching or licking at a wound or area of skin that is irritating him. Your vet will select the correct size for your cat.

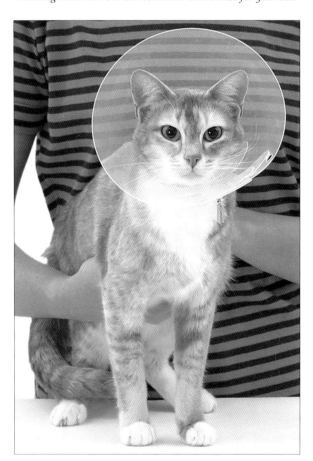

The following are all options that are commonly employed to prevent self-trauma.

Wound coverings

A variety of dressings, bandages and other coverings, including rigid casts, may be used to protect and to help in stabilizing a wound (see opposite).

'Elizabethan collars'

These are very effective devices for controlling self-trauma through licking and biting. If your cat needs to wear one, you must keep the collar clean. You should only remove it when you can watch your cat, as he may be able to inflict a surprising amount of damage on a wound even in a very short space of time.

You may also have to put up with bruises on the backs of your legs, caused by the brim of the collar being rammed against you as your cat rushes by!

'Anti-chew' preparations

These supposedly foul-tasting concoctions are applied to a cat's skin to discourage him from licking at any treated area. Such products do work with some cats, but others seem to like the taste or totally ignore it.

Distraction

If your cat is very well-behaved, you should be able to discourage him from interfering with a wound through discipline and distraction when you are with him.

As soon as he starts to show any interest in the wound, say 'NO' in a clear and stern voice in order to break his concentration, and then immediately offer him an alternative source of stimulation such as a toy.

Sedation

Some cats are so hyperactive that short-term sedation is the only way to enforce them to rest and to leave a wound alone. If your cat is such an individual, your vet will prescribe appropriate sedatives (see also page 94).

WARNING

When you are applying a bandage, or a piece of adhesive tape to secure the bandage, take great care not to put it on too tightly. Doing so may adversely affect the blood supply to the wound, and also to the part of your cat's body below the bandage.

DRESSINGS, BANDAGES AND CASTS

Appropriate dressings, bandages and rigid casts may be used for many reasons, including the following:

• To protect wounds from further injury, infection or self-trauma.

• To help in supporting and immobilizing orthopaedic conditions such as dislocations, painful joint sprains or fractures (see pages 44–6).

• To apply pressure in order to stop bleeding or to control swelling.

The care of any dressings, bandages or casts will involve the following:

• Protecting them from becoming wet and soiled.

• Preventing your cat from damaging or even removing them himself (all the techniques detailed opposite for protecting wounds are appropriate).

• Removing and replacing them: this will normally be carried out at your vet centre, but you may be asked to change a simple dressing in order to bathe a wound that requires frequent cleaning. You may also need to do so if your cat manages to remove or damage a dressing that has been applied at your vet centre.

Before attempting to change a bandage or dressing on your cat, make sure that your vet or veterinary nurse has given you the following:

• Precise instructions to follow.

• Any products – such as antibacterial solutions, creams, dressings and bandages – that you will need.

• A practical demonstration of what to do.

Changing a bandage or dressing

Before you go and get your cat, make sure that you are fully prepared. As well as new bandaging materials, you will need warm water, plenty of cotton wool, a towel, any antiseptic solutions, ointments and/or creams supplied by your vet centre, a pair of curved scissors (see page 115) and an assistant – changing a dressing on a cat is not a task to be undertaken single-handed. Cut a few strips of medical adhesive tape before you start, so that they will be ready to and hand when you need them.

1 Ask someone else to restrain your cat so that you have your hands free. For safety's sake, make sure that this person knows how to handle your cat properly (see pages 98–100).

2 Remove the existing bandage. It should be possible to unwrap this, but, if not, you will need to resort to the curved scissors.

3 Carefully unwrap any underlying padding and peel off any wound dressing. If either the padding or the dressing appears to be stuck to the wound, do

not pull at it, but moisten any adhered areas with warm water to loosen them.

4 Bathe the wound or affected area of skin and then re-dress it, following the instructions of your vet or veterinary nurse.

Bandaging a paw

Perhaps the most common type of wound covering is a paw bandage, and the vulnerable location of such bandages means that they often need changing because they easily become soiled or damaged. They are also the simplest of all bandages for a cat to remove!

If your cat accidentally damages a claw (see page 63) or cuts his paw, you may need to bandage it: this will protect the injury from further damage, and also make your cat more comfortable until you take him to be treated at your vet centre.

The technique outlined below can be adapted to the covering of other leg wounds.

1 Ask someone to restrain your cat for you. Clean an open wound by putting the paw into a bowl of warm, salty water or a special antiseptic solution. Keep changing the cleaning solution if it becomes contaminated with dirt. If at any time the wound starts to bleed, you should move on immediately to dressing and bandaging it.

2 Gently dry off the paw as much as you can, and cover over any bleeding or moist wound with impregnated gauze (this type of dressing should not stick to the wound).

3 Fill the gaps between your cat's toes with tiny wads of cotton wool, then wrap the whole paw twice with a generous amount of cotton wool peeled in one piece from the roll. This should reach about halfway up his foreleg and be about 2 cm (¾ in) thick, and will ensure that you do not put too much pressure on the skin when you apply the bandage.

4 Use a conforming bandage (see page 115) to wrap and compress the cotton wool. Wrap this backwards and forwards over the ends of your cat's toes, and then around his paw. Make sure that you leave a 'collar' of cotton wool at the top.

5 Repeat the process using a self-adhesive bandage (see page 115).

6 Use a length of medical adhesive tape to stick down the end of the bandage, being very careful not to apply this too tightly. As you apply the adhesive tape, wrap it loosely around the top of the bandage, so that it sticks to the bandage and also to your cat's fur: this will help to ensure that the bandage remains in position when your cat uses his paw.

Monitoring an ill cat

By diligently monitoring your cat's condition, you should quickly realize if he is not progressing as he should do. The nature and degree of monitoring that you need to carry out will depend on the seriousness of the illness or injury. Before you bring your cat home from your vet centre, find out what monitoring procedures you should undertake, and any specific signs that you will need to look out for in your cat's physical appearance or behaviour.

The following monitoring procedures are commonly carried out by veterinary nurses on their in-patients, and are relevant to nursing care at home.

Physical examinations

You should carry out a physical examination of your cat at least once a day. Any unexpected or abnormal features of his appearance may be a cause for concern, including the following:
- Dull, sunken or staring eyes
- Pale, dry gums
- The sudden appearance on his bedding or coat of blood or other discharges.
- An abnormal or foul smell associated with a wound, bandage or cast, with his body as a whole, or with his environment in general.
- An unexpected swelling associated with a wound.

Weighing

A decrease in your cat's weight during convalescence may be due to inadequate feeding or to dehydration (see pages 104–5), so regular and frequent weighing is an essential monitoring procedure.

You should weigh your cat at the same time of day on each occasion, as fluctuations that will occur in his body weight in each 24-hour period may otherwise be misleading. You may find it easiest to weigh your cat in his carrying basket, on a set of bathroom scales.

Behaviour monitoring

The most obvious signs of pain and discomfort shown by a cat include the following:
- Constant purring
- Sudden lethargy
- General dullness
- Reluctance to move
- Sudden mood changes
- Aggression when handled
- Restlessness

Inputs: food and water

It is essential to monitor accurately the water intake of a cat who is very ill, as any shortfalls must quickly be replaced by other means, such as by forced administration by mouth (see page 105) or directly into the blood via an intravenous drip at your vet centre (see page 93).

Adjustments to the cat's dietary regime will also need to be made if he fails to eat normally for more than a day or two (see page 104).

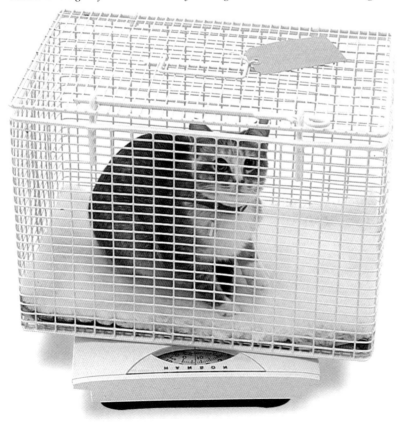

The simplest method for weighing your cat will be to put him on a set of bathroom scales, in his carrying basket, and then to deduct the weight of the basket and any bedding it contains.

Outputs: urine and faeces

By checking the approximate quantity and appearance of the urine that is produced by your cat during his convalescence, it will be possible to monitor his basic kidney function. The nature and quantity of any faeces produced will give a good indication of the condition of his digestive system.

If your vet wishes you to monitor your cat's urine production precisely, or to obtain samples for testing, he or she should provide a special false-bottomed litter-tray containing washable litter.

Body temperature

You may be asked to take your convalescing cat's temperature on a regular basis, to identify the first signs of fever development. The rectal temperature of a healthy cat is normally about 38.5°C (101.3°F).

Use the following technique to take your cat's temperature. You will need the help of an assistant to restrain him properly.

1 Check that the thermometer is re-set, cover its end with a lubricant jelly and then carefully insert it into the centre of your cat's anal ring by twisting it gently. Insert it sufficiently far that the tip is well through your cat's anal ring.

2 Holding on to the thermometer throughout, leave it in place for 30–60 seconds (follow the instructions for use accompanying your thermometer).

3 Gently remove the thermometer, and wipe it clean with cotton wool before reading off the recorded temperature and writing it down, along with the date and time taken.

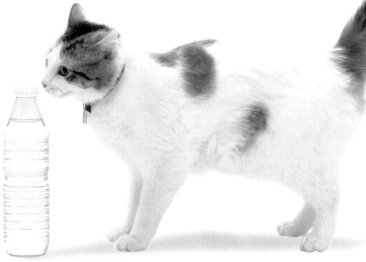

While your cat is convalescing, measure how much water he drinks each day. In the morning, fill his bowl to a set level. Over the next 24 hours, record how much you need to add to keep it at this level: the total will be the amount that your cat has drunk in that period.

When taking your cat's temperature, ask a helper to restrain him. Hold on to your cat's tail firmly – but not forcefully – with one hand, and hold the thermometer in the other.

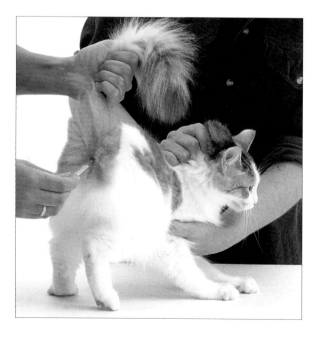

PULSE AND RESPIRATION RATES

A cat's pulse is taken on his inner thigh, close to his groin (this can be difficult to detect in some cats, and may be easier to feel directly through the chest wall). The pulse rate of a healthy cat at rest is normally between 110 and 140 beats per minute; the breathing rate is normally between 24 and 42 breaths per minute. An increase or decrease in either may be significant.

Preventive healthcare

If you are anything like me, you will never remember when you should be having your eyes tested or your tetanus vaccination updated, but now you have your cat's health to look after as well.

Some healthcare tasks – such as feeding – obviously need to be carried out daily, and not even I would need reminding to do those. However, other procedures – such as vaccination and worming – are required less frequently, and so are more likely to be overlooked.

The preventive-healthcare plan outlined here relates to a typical cross-bred cat living in the UK, and starts from the age of eight weeks – the age at which most kittens will move from their breeders to their new homes. Use this plan – together with the specific advice of your vet or a veterinary nurse – as a basis for creating a preventive-healthcare regime that is customized to your own cat: the more information that you add to it, the more useful it will become.

ROUTINE HEALTH-CHECKS

Taking your cat for veterinary check-ups, and carrying out routine health-checks at home, are both important aspects of preventive healthcare.

A kitten
With a vet • At eight, nine and 12 weeks, and at 12 months.
With a veterinary nurse • Physical-development and growth checks (ideally, every four weeks).
At home • Once a week, including weighing (see pages 8–9).

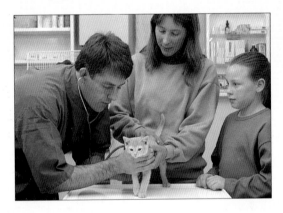

An adult cat
With a vet • Every 12 months; then from the age of 10 years, every six months.
At home • Once a week, including weighing (see pages 8–9).

PARASITE CONTROL

Worming against parasitic intestinal tapeworms and roundworms (see pages 28–9), and treating your cat and house for fleas (see pages 54–6).

Tapeworms
First dose • At eight weeks.
Subsequent doses • Every two to three months.

Roundworms
First dose • At eight weeks (a kitten's breeder should have wormed him at two-week intervals up to this age).
Second dose • At 10 weeks.
Third dose • At 12 weeks.
Subsequent doses • There is some debate among the veterinary profession as to how frequently kittens over the age of 12 weeks and adult cats should be wormed, but the majority of vets will recommend treating cats for roundworms every three months.

Flea prevention
(See also pages 54–6.)
Your cat • This will vary considerably, depending on the product used. A typical spray may be designed to be carried out every two weeks (but not before a kitten is 12 weeks old).
Your house • As well as routine vacuum-cleaning, you should spray your house with an appropriate product as often as directed.

DIET ALTERATION

You should change a kitten's diet from kitten food to adult cat food when he is 10–12 months old.

VACCINATIONS

Cat 'flu, feline panleucopenia and feline leukaemia virus infection (see pages 38–9 and 82–4).

A kitten
First vaccination • At nine weeks.
Second vaccination • At 12 weeks.
First booster • At 15 months.

An adult cat
Primary course • Two vaccinations, approximately two to four weeks apart.
Boosters • Every 12 months.

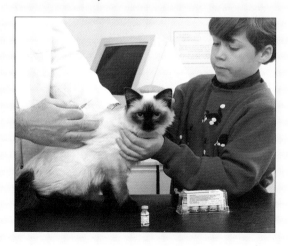

NEUTERING (SPAYING OR CASTRATION)

This should be carried out on all cats not intended for breeding at about six months of age.

TIMINGS OF TREATMENTS

The exact timing of certain procedures and events will vary, depending on factors such as the nature of the products used, the prevailing views of the veterinary profession in your country and the policy of your vet centre. Ask at your vet centre for further advice.

GROOMING

At home • Ideally, a quick groom daily, and a thorough groom weekly.
With a professional groomer • Every six months (for a long-haired cat).

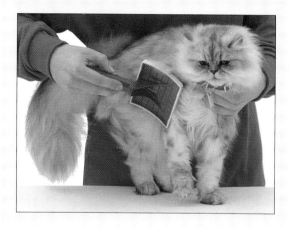

YOUR CAT'S DIARY

A record of your cat's individual anatomical quirks, together with other personal details, will be a very valuable document. Keeping a special diary updated can also become a project that many children and adults will find both entertaining and educational.

The diary should contain your cat's identification details and all relevant care information, including labels from his foods. It will also provide a good home for his medical cards – such as vaccination records – which are easy to mislay. You can customize your cat's diary by incorporating his healthcare plan into it (see above).

The more information you put into your cat's diary, the more valuable a resource it will become for you, the staff at your vet centre and anyone else who looks after your cat, such as the owner of his cattery.

Accidents and emergencies

This section of the book tells you how to cope with some of the most common accident-and-emergency situations in which your cat may be involved. You should familiarize yourself now with this information, so that in the event of an emergency you will be less likely to panic and of greater assistance to your cat.

Coping with an emergency

If your cat suddenly becomes ill or is badly injured in some way, it is very important that you try to stay calm. His life may be quite literally in your hands until your vet or a veterinary nurse can take over from you.

The step-by-step guides on the following pages give practical directions relating to some of the most common emergency situations to affect cats. Painful, but less critical, situations – such as lameness resulting from a thorn in a paw – are covered in relevant sections elsewhere in this book (refer to pages 10–11 for a guide to common conditions and associated symptoms).

What constitutes an emergency?

Those situations that are considered emergencies will vary from owner to owner. For example, a situation that may be taken as an emergency by an inexperienced owner may be less cause for concern to someone who has lived with cats for years. However, some accidents and illnesses are obvious emergencies to all.

An emergency is any situation affecting your cat that you believe may be causing him undue pain, or placing his life in danger. If you are unsure as to whether or not your cat needs immediate medical attention, it is much better to be over-cautious and to contact your vet centre for advice. Your vet or a veterinary nurse will be able to give you precise instructions over the telephone as to what actions you should take (see page 90), and, if you are worrying unnecessarily, will put your mind at rest.

What to do first

If your cat has an accident and is injured in any way, or if he suddenly shows what you interpret as serious symptoms of illness, contact your vet centre as soon as you can. You should only delay this in order to carry out resuscitation techniques, or to deal with any

immediately life-threatening situations such as severe bleeding. Ideally, you should stay with your cat and carry out first aid while somebody else makes the call.

The staff at your vet centre will give you specific instructions. Do not demand that your vet visits you, but let him or her decide what is the most appropriate course of action to take. If your cat can be moved, and you are able and willing to move him (see page 117), your vet is very likely to suggest that you take your cat straight to the vet centre so that he can benefit as quickly as possible from its facilities.

Dealing with a cat in pain

A cat's natural instinct when he is either frightened or in pain will be to run away from whatever he thinks may be causing the fear or pain. As a result, many injured cats are very shy and suspicious of people – including their owners. It is not unusual, for instance, for a cat with a broken leg to disappear from the scene of an accident altogether.

In a such a situation, your instinct may be to chase after your cat to catch him, so that you can help him. However, by doing so – especially with other people – you are likely to frighten him even more.

If your cat is involved in an accident, he may manage to struggle home despite his injuries, and may then find somewhere safe to curl up and hide. Wherever he is – indoors or out – you will need to find him. You are most likely to be successful if you do the following:

1 Call your cat's name in order to try to identify where he is, and listen carefully for any response that he may make. Remember that a cat who is in severe pain will often purr continuously.

2 Keep talking to him in a calm and friendly voice.

3 If he is outdoors, organize any helpers that you have to form a large circle around your cat: their presence may discourage him from making an escape.

4 If possible, make sure that you have something in which to put your cat (ideally, his carrying basket, but a cardboard box will do), or something in which to wrap him (such as a large towel, or a coat: see page 100), in case he becomes aggressive.

5 When you find your cat, get down to his level and talk to him. Only move closer when he seems calm, and, if he looks anxious and flighty, stop moving.

6 When you reach your cat, he may let you stroke him. However, if he is in pain he may resent being

EMERGENCY CHECKLIST

In any emergency situation, your first priorities should be to do the following in the most appropriate order:

• Apprehend your cat if he is free (see left), and if necessary prevent him from escaping by putting him in his carrying basket or a suitable cardboard box. Keep any noise to a minimum and the light dim (if necessary, place a blanket over your cat's basket or box to cut out the light); this should encourage him to remain calm.

• Carry out any essential first-aid procedures that may save your cat's life or reduce his pain before he receives professional veterinary attention (see pages 116–17).

• Contact your vet centre for specific advice, or to arrange for assistance.

• Keep your cat warm by wrapping him in a foil blanket or bubble-wrap, and place heat-generating pads next to his body, if you have your first-aid kit (see below).

• Unless it is imperative to move your cat for safety – for example, away from a road or to prevent him from escaping – only do this if you are sure that it is safe, or if you are advised to do so by your veterinary staff.

• Prevent your cat from injuring you or anyone else.

Your first-aid kit

It is a good idea to have a first-aid kit for your cat. Commercially made kits are available but, in my view, these often do not contain some of the most important items that you will need in an emergency.

My advice is to make up your own first-aid kit, with the help of your vet or a veterinary nurse. Take the kit everywhere that you visit with your cat, and make sure that all the family know when and how to use it.

A good first-aid kit should include the following:

1 Sheet of bubble-wrap
2 Cotton wool
3 Moist face-wipes
4 Adhesive bandages
5 Conforming bandage
6 Disposable gloves
7 Veterinary antiseptic
8 5 ml and 10 ml syringes
9 Foil blanket
10 Washing-soda (sodium carbonate) crystals (see page 120)
11 Salt (for bathing wounds)
12 Large towel
13 Spare collars
14 Heat-generating pads
15 Impregnated gauze
16 Sterile dressings
17 Thermometer
18 Curved, round-ended scissors
19 Long-handled, fine tweezers
20 Magnifying glass
21 Small torch and spare batteries
22 Small pliers
23 Pen-knife

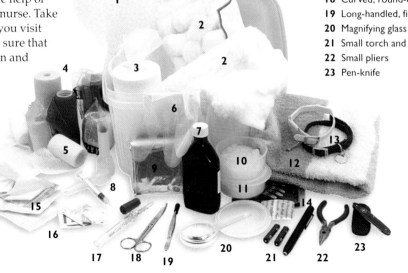

touched at all, and may lash out at you with his claws, so you must be extremely careful.

7 If your cat seems calm and you are used to handling him, gain his confidence and then quickly seize him by the scruff of his neck (see pages 99–100). Lift him off the ground by his scruff so that he cannot squirm around and injure you with his hind claws, then quickly put him into his carrying basket or a box. If your cat is being aggressive and you do not feel confident about the scruffing technique, cover him with a towel or a coat – using this to protect your hands – and 'smother' him in your arms so that he cannot wriggle free. If you cannot get close to your cat, or you are concerned that injuries could be made worse through handling, wait for help to arrive.

8 If you do catch your cat, quickly move him indoors or even to a car so that he cannot escape, before taking him out of his basket to assess his condition further or carry out any first-aid procedures. If possible, ask an assistant to help you to restrain him properly (see pages 98–100). If your cat was difficult to catch, it is unlikely that you will have to carry out life-saving first aid. In this case, your priority should be to get him to your vet centre as soon as possible.

Organizing others

Try to organize the help of at least one other person when dealing with an emergency involving your cat. That person can telephone your vet centre while you stay with your cat, and another pair of hands will make handling him and first-aid procedures easier and safer.

No matter how many other people are keen to help, stay in control and tell them what you wish them to do. You will then be able to turn the hindrance of casual bystanders into practical help.

PREVENTING ACCIDENTS

By being a safety-conscious owner, you may be able to prevent your cat from becoming involved in some of the most common accident-and-emergency situations. Remember the following points:

• Be aware of hazards in your home and garden, such as trailing wires, medicines, open garden sheds, open washing-machine or tumble-drier doors and rubbish bins.

• Do not leave your cat with small toys or other objects that he could pick up in his mouth and swallow.

• Never carry your cat in your arms outdoors, other than in your garden, and only then if it is safe for him to run off if he jumps free.

• If your cat is near an open window that is high off the ground, or sitting on the edge of a balcony, do not try to grab him, as he may jump away from you. Instead, try to tempt him down or indoors.

A ROAD ACCIDENT

1 Ask another person – if someone is available – to warn approaching traffic of the accident.

2 Ask someone to telephone a vet centre.

3 If your cat is conscious and able to move, approach him very quietly and slowly (see page 115).

4 If he has collapsed and appears to be unconscious, check whether or not he is breathing by watching his chest for movement. If you are in any doubt, pluck a small tuft of fur from his coat and hold it directly in front of his nostrils.

5 If your cat is not breathing, check that his airway is clear. Open his mouth and look right down to the back of his throat. Remove any obvious obstructions and pull his tongue forward.

6 If there is no obvious obstruction, extend your cat's neck by lifting up his chin and then, with his mouth closed, give him mouth-to-nose artificial respiration. Do this by taking a breath and then breathing out a little air into your cat's nostrils: his rib cage should just rise. Repeat at about 30 breaths per minute.

Try to feel for your cat's heartbeat by holding your fingers firmly against his chest, just behind his left elbow. As with other techniques, you should practise doing this so that you will know how to locate your cat's heartbeat in an emergency.

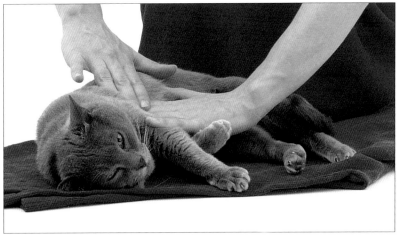

7 Between breaths, check for a heartbeat (see opposite, below). Alternatively, feel for a pulse by pressing your fingers against the top of his inner thigh.

8 If you are absolutely sure that your cat's heart has stopped, begin chest compressions (DO NOT do this if there is a chance that your cat has fractured ribs or another chest injury). To carry out the compressions, apply intermittent pressure in a 'cough-like' manner, with two fingers of each hand placed flat on either side of your cat's chest, just behind his elbows. Do this at a rate of two per second. Every four compressions, give your cat artificial respiration for two breaths. Keep checking for a heartbeat or pulse, and only stop compressing your cat's chest when you feel a consistent pulse, or when veterinary help arrives.

9 If your cat is bleeding, apply pressure to the apparent source of any haemorrhage. If you have your first-aid kit with you, bind a large pad of cotton wool firmly to the affected area with a conforming bandage. Otherwise, use a piece of clothing and apply the necessary pressure with your hands. If blood soaks through, do not remove the dressing (you may disrupt any clots that have formed) but simply apply another dressing on top.

10 Cover any other open wounds to prevent them from becoming contaminated with dirt. If a skin wound has broken bones protruding through it, apply a doughnut-shaped ring-pad dressing made from a bandage, scarf or other item as follows:
  • Wind the bandage around your hand three times to form a ring shape.
  • Take the bandage off your hand and then wind the rest of it around the circle. Tuck in the end securely, and smooth out any wrinkles.

11 If your cat appears to have a broken leg and you have no choice but to move him, be extremely careful about how you carry him (see above, right). If he is still conscious and could struggle when you move him, splint the leg first if possible. A tightly rolled newspaper or a piece of wood will make a suitable temporary splint. Place this against the affected limb, on the opposite side to any open wound, and then bandage it firmly in place.

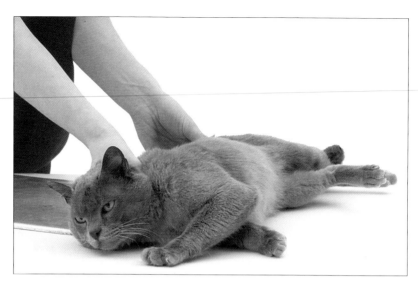

To move an injured cat on to a makeshift stretcher – such as a sheet of plywood or a metal tray – grasp the fur at his scruff and lower back, and then gently slide him on to the stretcher.

Moving an injured cat

In a carrying basket • By far the best way to move an injured cat is in a proper carrying basket that is large enough for him to lie down in. The next best option is a large, sturdy cardboard box.

Making a stretcher • If you do not have a carrying basket or a box, make a stretcher from a piece of wood or other rigid object, such as a large road atlas. Lie this next to your cat, then slide him on to it by grasping handfuls of fur along his back. Another option is to make a sling using a blanket or sheet.

Carrying your cat • If you are on your own, and your cat is not too badly injured, you may have to carry him. Grasp the scruff of his neck with one hand so that you have control of his head. Place the palm of your free hand under his chest, between his forelegs, and then scoop his body up under your forearm.

WARNING

If your cat is unable to lie in an upright position, with his head up, do not move him unless absolutely necessary (for instance, to get him away from a road). If he has any spinal injuries, moving him could cause further damage, so wait for veterinary assistance to arrive.

Never give an injured cat anything by mouth, in case he requires surgery (see page 94).

A SEVERE SKIN WOUND

1   If the wound contains one or more foreign bodies and is bleeding, attempt to remove any object that may be driven deeper into the wound by a pressure dressing, and then apply a dressing of this type as quickly as possible (see step 9, page 117). Bright-red blood spurting from the wound is a sure indication that an artery has been severed. Apply pressure immediately to the source of the spurt, using your finger. If possible, keep it there for 10 minutes, or immediately apply a pressure dressing.

• If the wound is not bleeding, leave any foreign bodies alone, or you may cause further damage and bleeding in trying to remove them. Instead, apply a ring-pad dressing around the entire wound (see step 10, page 117).

• If a large foreign body is protruding a long way through the skin, carefully bandage around it.

2   If the wound does not appear to contain any foreign bodies, but is bleeding, apply a pressure dressing (see step 9, page 117).

3   If the wound does not appear to contain any foreign bodies and is not bleeding, gently bathe it with a veterinary antiseptic solution and then carefully dry off the area. Apply a protective dressing using impregnated gauze wrapped with plenty of cotton wool, compressed with a conforming bandage. If at any stage of the cleaning and washing procedure the wound begins to bleed, stop and apply a pressure dressing (see step 9, page 117).

4   If you can move your cat and you think that it is safe to do so, take him to your vet centre as soon as possible; otherwise, wait for your vet to arrive.

COLLAPSE

If your cat appears to be unconscious and is totally unaware of your presence, do the following:

1   Check whether he is breathing (see step 4, page 116). If he is not breathing, check his throat for foreign bodies or swellings. If none is obvious, begin artificial respiration (see step 6, page 116).

2   Check for a heartbeat or pulse. If there is none, begin chest compressions (see steps 7–8, page 117).

3   Contact your vet centre as soon as possible.

4   If your cat is conscious, keep him calm, quiet and warm while you wait for help to arrive.

BREATHING DIFFICULTY OR CHOKING

1   Immediately look inside your cat's mouth for any obvious foreign body. DO NOT poke about in his mouth without looking, or you may push a foreign body back into his throat.

2   If there is a foreign body in the mouth, attempt to remove it (use the tweezers in your first-aid kit if appropriate). However, if the object appears to be deep in your cat's throat, leave it alone or you may push it further down towards his airway.

3   If your cat is choking, quickly lift him up by his hindlegs so that his head is dangling down, and slap the side of his rib cage with two fingers of your free hand, in sharp, 'cough-like', jerky movements. You should only move your hands a little, in order to stimulate a sudden rush of air from his lungs: this should help to dislodge any foreign body stuck at the back of the throat. Be sensible about the amount of pressure that you apply, particularly with a kitten.

4   As soon as your cat coughs out the foreign body, settle him on the ground and let him calm down in his own time.

5   If your cat has a cat flap, lock it, and ensure that he cannot leave the house by any other exit.

6   Continue to watch over your cat. Be careful not to stimulate him in any way, and try to discourage him from moving about.

7   Contact your vet centre to tell your vet what has happened. There is little point in doing so sooner (unless you have someone with you who can make a telephone call), as this will waste precious time: your cat's best chance of survival rests with you.

A bandage like this one, used to apply pressure to a bleeding wound on a cat's back, could cut off the blood supply to his forelegs if it were applied too tightly. Use your common sense when using any type of bandage on your cat's body.

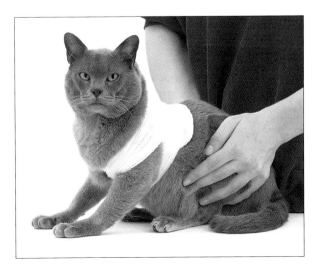

LACK OF CO-ORDINATION

(See also seizures [below] strange behaviour [page 122] and heatstroke [page 123].)

1 If your cat has a cat flap, lock it.
2 Stop your cat from moving around by confining him to his carrying basket or to a cardboard box.
3 Leave him in a darkened, quiet room (or cover his basket or box with a blanket, to keep out the light), and stay with him.
4 Contact your vet centre.

A SEIZURE (CONVULSION OR 'FIT')

1 If your cat is indoors, darken the room and keep the area quiet.
2 Contact your vet centre.
3 If your cat has a cat flap, lock it.
4 Stay with your cat, but do not touch him unless he is about to injure himself. In this case, move him carefully so as to stimulate him as little as possible.
5 Even if you think that your cat may be choking on his tongue or about to bite it, do not handle his mouth: he may bite you by accident.
6 Your cat should stop fitting after a few minutes. Continue to watch him, but do not move him or encourage him to move by himself. If he does get up, do not try to stop him, as your restraint may stimulate him to have another seizure.
7 If your cat continues to fit, keep observing him and wait for your vet to arrive.

SUDDEN, SEVERE VOMITING

(See also pages 26–7.)

1 Restrict your cat to one room.
2 If he has a cat flap, lock it.
3 Do not let him eat or drink.
4 Contact your vet centre.
5 Each time your cat vomits, note down the time, and the consistency of the vomit. This may help your vet to identify the cause of the problem.

A good way to keep your cat warm when he is ill or has been injured is to cover him with bubble-wrap.

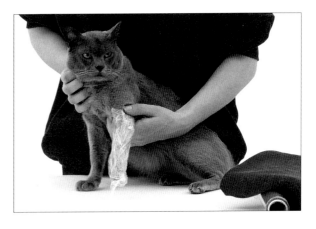

Having cooled down an area of burned skin under plenty of cold running water, cover the affected part with cling film. This will protect the wound and help to prevent fluid loss, without adhering to the raw tissue.

SUDDEN, SEVERE DIARRHOEA

(See also pages 32–3).

1 Restrict your cat to one room, with a litter-tray.
2 Make sure that he does not eat.
3 Contact your vet centre.
4 Each time your cat passes diarrhoea, note down the time, and the consistency and quantity of what he produces. This information may help your vet to identify the cause of the problem.

A HEAT BURN

1 Immediately cool down the affected area of your cat's skin by thoroughly soaking it with very cold, running water for at least 10 minutes. While doing this, contact your vet centre.
2 Cover the area with cling film, then wrap your cat to keep him warm. If you have a foil blanket or bubble-wrap (see page 115), use this with heat-generating pads.

A CHEMICAL BURN

1 Prevent your cat from trying to groom himself, as he may transfer the chemical to his mouth.
2 Wash the affected area of skin under copious amounts of cold running water. While you are doing this, contact your vet centre.

INGESTION OF A POSSIBLE POISON

If you know or think that your cat may have ingested a poisonous substance, contact your vet centre as soon as you have carried out initial and appropriate emergency care (see below). If your cat has a cat flap, lock it. DO NOT attempt to make your cat vomit unless there is a clear indication to do so – if in doubt, don't.

If possible, tell your vet the name of the substance that your cat has swallowed. If he or she is not familiar with it, a veterinary nurse may be able to find out more information about it while you are on your way to the vet centre. Take the product packaging with you.

Corrosive acids

Examples include sulphuric acid (in car batteries), hydrochloric acid (in some kettle descalers) and nitric acid (in some household cleaners).

Administer a dilute solution of bicarbonate of soda (2.5 ml [half a teaspoonful] in 250 ml [8 fl oz] of water) by mouth – ideally, using a syringe (see page 105) – to help to neutralize the corrosive chemical. Try to administer about 5–10 ml (1–2 teaspoonfuls) of this solution. DO NOT try to make your cat vomit.

Corrosive alkalis

Examples include caustic soda (used in some paint strippers), oven-cleaning chemicals, tar and creosote.

Administer vinegar (diluted 50:50 with water) or orange juice by mouth – ideally, using a syringe (see page 105) – to help to neutralize the chemical. Try to administer about 5–10 ml (1–2 teaspoonfuls) to your cat. DO NOT try to make him vomit.

Irritants

Examples include decaying meat, plants (dumb cane, poinsettia, laburnum, daffodil bulbs), lead (in golf balls, putty, old linoleum, paraffin), arsenic (in some insecticides) and mercury (in some moss-killers). DO NOT try to make your cat vomit.

Narcotics

Examples include barbiturates, turpentine and paraffin.
1 If you see your cat eat a narcotic substance, try to make him vomit immediately (see above, right). However, if you think that your cat may have eaten a narcotic substance, but you did not see him do it and he now appears to be sedated, DO NOT try to make him vomit: there is a possibility that his swallow reflex may be affected, and he could inhale his vomit.
2 Constantly stimulate your cat, to try to prevent him from falling asleep.

MAKING YOUR CAT VOMIT

To induce vomiting, place a few crystals of washing soda (sodium carbonate) on the back of your cat's tongue or, if you do not have any washing soda available, administer a strong salt or mustard solution to him by mouth.

(Note: a cat's stomach will normally have emptied in a few hours, so there is no point in trying to make your cat vomit if you suspect that he may have swallowed a poisonous substance more than four hours earlier.)

Convulsants

Examples include slug bait (metaldehyde), anti-freeze (ethylene glycol), laurel leaves, lead, strychnine (in some mole-killers). Chocolate can also be very harmful to a cat if it is eaten in excess.

If you see your cat consume a convulsant substance, try to make him vomit immediately (see above).

SEVERE LAMENESS
1 If your cat has a cat flap, lock it.
2 If he cannot bear any weight on the affected leg, or if it looks an unusual shape or appears very swollen, contact your vet centre immediately.
3 Confine your cat to his carrying basket.
4 If he will not keep the affected leg still, splint it (see page 117).
5 If he can bear can weight on the affected leg, refer to page 47 for further advice.

It is well worth learning a few simple bandaging techniques: for example, it is possible to make a very strong support for a broken leg from nothing more rigid than cotton wool and conforming bandages, as shown below. Ask your vet or a nurse to show you how to carry out techniques such as this.

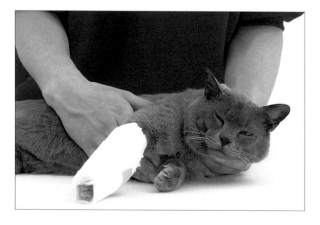

To control a skin swelling, hold a bag of frozen peas, or some ice cubes wrapped in a cloth, over the affected area. Use the same technique on a swollen or painful sprained joint.

APPARENT PARALYSIS

1 If your cat does not appear to be able to stand up, or can only raise his front end off the ground, you must contact your vet centre immediately.
2 Stay with your cat and keep him calm, quiet and warm. Do not attempt to move him.

A SUDDEN, SEVERE SKIN SWELLING

Although a subcutaneous abscess may seem to develop overnight as a result of a puncture wound sustained during a cat fight (see pages 60–1), an adverse reaction to an insect sting or bite may become obvious on a cat's skin within a matter of minutes.

Due to a wasp or bee sting

1 If the sting is in your cat's mouth, nose or throat you must seek veterinary attention immediately, as any swelling may block his airway.
2 If your cat has been stung by a bee, the sting may still be in the skin. If you can see it, carefully grasp it close to the skin, using tweezers, and remove it.
3 Help to neutralize the effects of a bee sting by gently bathing the affected area with a solution made up of 10 ml (1 dessertspoonful) of bicarbonate of soda to 600 ml (1 pint) of water. For a wasp sting, use vinegar diluted 50:50 with water as a bathing solution. If neither of these substances is available, bathing the affected area with soap and water should help to relieve the pain of the sting.

WARNING

Never attempt to remove any type of foreign body – either manually or with any instrument such as a pair of tweezers – from your cat's eye. You could cause further damage, especially if your cat were to move suddenly.

4 Apply a cold compress, such as a cloth wetted with very cold water (packed with ice if possible) or a bag of frozen peas, to try to control the swelling.

Due to an unknown cause

(See also pages 47 and 60–1.)
1 If your cat has a cat flap and he is indoors, lock it.
2 Apply a cold compress, such as a cloth dampened with very cold water (packed with ice if possible), or a bag of frozen peas, to try to control the extent of the swelling.
3 Contact your vet centre.

AN EYE INJURY

1 Prevent your cat from rubbing or scratching at his eye: by doing so, he is likely to cause further damage.
2 Look closely for any foreign body – such as a piece of stalk or grit – that may be trapped behind your cat's upper or lower eyelid. Using a magnifying glass may help. If you can see a foreign body, try to flush it out by pouring warm water gently over the affected eye. However, if doing this causes your cat further distress, stop immediately.
3 Contact your vet centre.
4 If the eye is swollen, apply a compress in the form of a cloth wetted with very cold water.

If your cat's eye is bleeding, gently cover it over with a pad of cotton wool until your vet can examine the eye. If blood starts to seep through this pad, place another one on top.

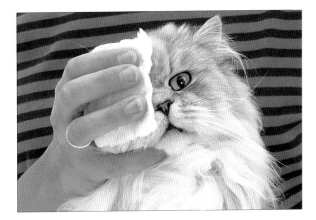

COAT CONTAMINATION

(See also a chemical burn on page 120.)
Whatever the kind of coat contamination, first check the underlying skin for burns and treat as necessary (see page 120). Contact your vet centre immediately if your cat's skin looks inflamed, if you are unable to remove the contaminant successfully, if you think he may have ingested some of the substance contaminating his coat, or if he is unwell in any other way.

Non-oily compounds

An example is a disinfectant solution.
  Wash the affected area of your cat's coat with copious amounts of water. DO NOT use any form of detergent, as this may increase the speed with which any toxic chemical is absorbed through the skin.

Liquid oily compounds

Examples are engine oil and creosote.
1 Smear the affected area with a commercial hand-cleaning jelly, or with liquid paraffin or cooking oil.
2 Wash the affected coat with a detergent, such as washing-up liquid, and plenty of warm water. Rinse thoroughly, then repeat as many times as necessary. DO NOT use petrol or other inflammable liquid.

Solid oily compounds

An example is tar.
1 If possible, carefully clip off the contaminated hair.
2 Alternatively, rub commercial hand-cleaning jelly, liquid paraffin or cooking oil into the affected area, then treat as for a liquid oily compound (see above).

FOREIGN BODIES

Always stop to think before rushing to remove a foreign body, or you could make matters worse for your cat.

Gagging

1 If your cat has a cat flap, lock it.
2 If your cat cannot close his mouth properly, if he is drooling excessively or if he appears to be gagging, immediately wrap him in a towel to restrain him (see page 100) and look inside his mouth.
3 If you can see a foreign body, only attempt to remove it if you are sure that doing so will not cause any further damage, and that you will not dislodge it and accidentally push it further towards the back of your cat's throat. DO NOT try to remove a fishing hook or other sharp object that may be lodged in the lining of his mouth or throat.
4 Contact your vet centre as soon as possible.

A foreign body in the nose

1 If your cat has a cat flap, lock it.
2 If you see a foreign body protruding from one of your cat's nostrils, DO NOT attempt to remove it. The object may be longer than you think, and by trying to remove it you may inadvertently break it off inside your cat's nose.
3 Contact your vet centre.

Violent head-shaking

If your cat is shaking his head violently, he may well have a foreign body in his ear. DO NOT put anything into his ear hole.
1 If he has a cat flap, lock it.
2 Contact your vet centre immediately.

A swallowed foreign body

(See also page 30.)
1 If your cat has a cat flap, lock it.
2 Make sure that your cat does not eat or drink.
3 Contact your vet centre immediately.

A foreign body in the anus

1 If your cat has a cat flap, lock it.
2 Examine the foreign body closely. If it looks sharp, leave it alone. Otherwise, wrap your cat in a towel to restrain him (see page 100), then grasp the foreign body with a pair of tweezers and gently pull it. If there is any resistance at all, stop immediately.
3 Contact your vet centre.

STRANGE BEHAVIOUR

(See also lack of co-ordination on page 119.)
1 Examine your cat to see if there is anything obvious that may be wrong with him physically.
2 Try to identify anything unusual in his environment that may be upsetting him.
3 Contact your vet centre for advice.
4 If possible, it is a good idea to videotape your cat's behaviour, as he may not behave in the same way once he gets to your vet centre.

A BROKEN TOOTH

Although a cat with a broken tooth (or teeth) may continue to eat normally, do not believe that this is not a painful condition: it is. It can also lead to infection (see pages 22–4). If you notice a broken tooth in your cat's mouth, contact your vet centre straight away.

BLEEDING FROM THE MOUTH

1 If your cat has a cat flap, lock it.
2 Carefully examine your cat's mouth and tongue in an attempt to discover the source of the blood.
3 If you identify a foreign body, only attempt to remove it if it is not stuck into the gums, tongue or cheeks. If you can see a foreign body, but think that you cannot or should not try to remove it, or there is another obvious but unidentifiable cause of the bleeding, contact your vet centre immediately.
4 If the quantity of blood is small and there is no obvious cause of it, keep your cat calm and quiet. Monitor him for the next 10 minutes. If the bleeding does not stop, or worsens, contact your vet centre.

STRAINING TO PASS URINE

(See also pages 66–7.)
If your cat is straining but is not passing any urine at all, lock his cat flap and then contact your vet centre as a matter of urgency.

STRAINING TO PASS FAECES

1 If your cat has a cat flap, lock it.
2 Contact your vet centre.
3 Try to distract your cat from continually straining, as he may cause further problems (see also page 31).

SUDDEN ABDOMINAL SWELLING

Keep your cat indoors and seek veterinary attention immediately.

HEATSTROKE

If your cat is suffering from heatstroke, he will be restless, distressed and will pant continually. As his condition worsens, he will start to drool excessively and become unsteady on his feet.
1 Cool your cat down immediately using cold-water baths or by soaking him with running water.

If your think that your cat may be suffering from heatstroke, you should immerse him in a basin of cold water and then wrap him with soaked towels or blankets to bring down his temperature.

WARNING

If your cat gets into trouble in water, but you are not a strong swimmer or the water conditions are hazardous, do not risk your life in order to save him.

---

2 Cover him with soaked towels or blankets, and continue to douse him with water.
3 Contact your vet centre immediately.

DROWNING

1 If you are able to rescue your cat, immediately turn him upside-down to help to drain the water from his lungs. Hold him up and off the ground by his hindlegs, and swing his body from side to side.
2 If your cat is not breathing, start artificial respiration (see step 6, page 116). Between breaths, check for a heartbeat or pulse. If you cannot detect either, begin chest compressions at the same time (see steps 7–8, pages 116–17). If your cat fails to start breathing on his own, continue with the artificial respiration and chest compressions until a vet can take over.
3 Contact the nearest vet centre as soon as possible. If you are alone, call out to attract the attention of someone who can help.
4 If your cat begins to cough, splutter and then to breathe on his own, dry off as much water as you can and keep him warm.

AN ELECTRIC SHOCK

1 Switch off the electricity.
2 If your cat is not breathing, begin artificial respiration (see step 6, page 116). Between breaths, check for a heartbeat or pulse. If you cannot feel either, start chest compressions at the same time (see steps 7–8, pages 116–17).
3 Contact a vet centre as soon as possible. If you are on your own, call out to attract the attention of someone to help.
4 Continue trying to resuscitate your cat until he begins to breathe by himself or veterinary help arrives.
5 If your cat is breathing, or if you resuscitate him, treat any burns (see page 119) and keep him warm.

The end of your cat's life

Your cat may be an independent soul, but he is a member of your family, and you and all those who have shared his life will be devastated when he dies. Before you come to terms with your loss, you will inevitably ride an emotional roller-coaster that may take you through stages of shock and disbelief, sadness, anger, yearning and depression. In your mind, you will relive many events from your cat's life, including those immediately prior to his death.

When he is gone, you will miss him more than you could ever have imagined possible. However, it is very important, particularly for the sake of any children you may have, that you handle your cat's death so as to minimize the grief that you all feel and to maximize the fond memories of your relationship.

EUTHANASIA

Your cat may die suddenly and unexpectedly as a result of an accident or acute illness, or he may be fortunate enough to pass away quietly in his sleep when he is a happy old man.

However, if your cat is terminally ill and is suffering unnecessarily – even if he is still young – you must be brave enough to do the right thing, and to ask your vet to put your cat out of his misery by ending his life quickly and humanely through euthanasia.

What is euthanasia?

Often referred to as 'putting a cat to sleep', euthanasia is the painless, premature ending of a cat's life to prevent him from continuing to suffer from the pain, discomfort and misery of terminal illness or injury. It can only be carried out by a vet, and normally involves injecting a lethal dose of an anaesthetic drug directly into a cat's bloodstream through a leg vein, in the same way as a general anaesthetic is administered (see pages 94–5).

The cat will lose consciousness and die within seconds of the injection being given: all he will feel is the slight scratch of the needle penetrating his skin.

Deciding on euthanasia

The decision to euthanase your cat is one that you should make together with all the members of your family and your vet. Before making a decision one way or the other about your cat's future, you should be fully aware of the seriousness of his condition and of all the options that are open.

The following are the kinds of questions to which you should obtain clear and precise answers:
• What is wrong with my cat?
• Is he in pain?
• Will he recover?
• What could be done to help control his symptoms?
• What quality of life would this treatment give him?
• What kind of nursing will he need?

Your cat's condition may be such that euthanasia is clearly the only option open, but most owners of terminally ill cats are faced with a more difficult decision. Your vet will of course give you his or her recommendation as to which course of action is most appropriate, but the final decision must be yours.

Taking your time

Unless your cat's present condition dictates otherwise (for instance, if he is seriously injured in an accident), do not feel pressurized to make an immediate decision about his future. It is important that you consider carefully everything that your vet has told you, and that you discuss all the options as a family.

For each option, think what your cat's quality of life will be. Will he be really living, or simply existing?

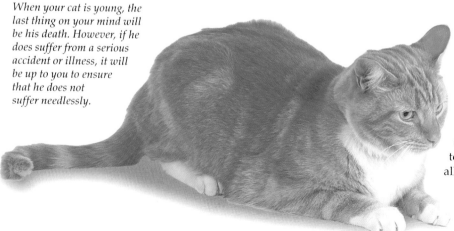

When your cat is young, the last thing on your mind will be his death. However, if he does suffer from a serious accident or illness, it will be up to you to ensure that he does not suffer needlessly.

Try as hard as you can to ignore your own feelings: you must do what is right for your cat. Many owners later regret having kept their terminally ill cats alive because they could not bear to say goodbye.

If you cannot reach a decision, ask any cat-owning friends and relatives for their opinions, as they should be able to consider your cat's condition from a more detached perspective. Take the time that you need. If you decide to euthanase your cat and you feel confident that you have made the correct decision, you will be much less likely to complicate and compound your grief through feelings of guilt.

What happens next?

If you decide that euthanasia is the right option to take, your vet or a veterinary nurse will help you to make the necessary practical arrangements.

Your cat's euthanasia can be carried out by your vet either at your vet centre, or in your own home: the decision should be up to you. My personal feeling is that it is most appropriate for a cat to die at home, in familar surroundings.

Who should be there?

Only you as a family can make that decision. Very rarely are there any complications in euthanasia, but you should be aware that – if your cat's circulation is very poor – it may be difficult for your vet to locate a suitable vein in which to administer the injection. Some owners prefer to leave the room while the procedure is carried out, but choose to return afterwards to see their cats at peace and free from pain.

Saying goodbye

No matter where your cat is euthanased, or whether you will be present, all the family should try to say a final goodbye, as this will help you to cope with your sense of loss. When, where and how you do so is up to you. Some owners prefer to say goodbye to their cats before they are euthanased; others may find it easier and more appropriate to hold some kind of simple ceremony that is meaningful to them.

AFTER YOUR CAT'S DEATH

Whether your cat dies naturally or through euthanasia, you will have to decide what to do with his body. If you would like to bury him in your garden or in some other special place, you should check first with your local environmental-health authority that you are allowed to do so. It may be possible where you live to bury your cat in a special pet cemetery.

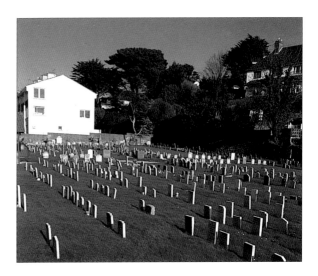

Cemeteries for pets are now commonplace in some countries. Their existence is proof enough that cats hold a very special place in our lives, even long after they have died.

Cremation

Most owners choose to have their cats cremated: your vet centre should be able to arrange this. Many owners have the ashes returned, so that they can bury them or dispose of them in one of their cats' favourite haunts.

One young family, whose cat had been confined indoors for the last years of his life because of illness, took his ashes out into the garden and simply scattered them in the breeze. When he was alive, the cat had spent hours sitting at the window, gazing out into the garden, and at last they had been able to set him free. By doing so, they also took a vital step in coping with their grief at his loss.

Even if you decide not to have your cat's ashes returned, you and your family may like to hold some kind of ceremony to celebrate your cat's life: planting a tree or shrub in his memory may make you feel better.

BEREAVEMENT COUNSELLORS

If you find that you are not coping very well with your cat's death and that your sadness is affecting other areas of your life, you must talk to someone who understands what you are going through. Contact your vet centre, and speak to your vet or to a veterinary nurse whom you know well. He or she may decide to put you in touch with a bereavement counsellor, who will be able to help you to come to terms with your loss.

Index

ACKNOWLEDGEMENTS

The publishing of any book is a team effort, and I would like to express my sincere thanks to the many organizations and to the individuals – both human and feline – who have played a part in creating *Cat Doctor*.

I am particularly indebted to the following friends and colleagues for their general advice and guidance, and for their specific contributions:

David Ashworth BVetMed MRCVS

Serena Brownlie Phd BVMS CertSAC MRCVS

Steve Butterworth MA VetMB CertVR DSAO MRCVS

Elspeth Down BVetMed MRCVS

John Down BVetMed MRCVS

Hugh Duffin BVetMed MRCVS

Jonathan Elliot NA VetMB Phd CertSAC MRCVS

Gary England BVetMed Phd DVR CertVA MRCVS

Maxine Field VN

Peter Holt BVMS Phd CBiol DipECVS MIBiol FRCVS

Janet & Craig Irvine-Smith BVSc (Pret) MRCVS and all the staff of the Stonehenge Veterinary Hospital.

Morag Kerr BVMS BSc Phd MRCVS

Richard Laven BVetMed MRCVS

Andrew Lawley BSc BVetMed MRCVS

Ben Linnell BVetMed MRCVS

Chris Little BVMA Phd Cert SAC MRCVS

Joanna Morris BSc BVetMed MRCVS

Sue Oxley VN

Simon Petersen-Jones DVetMed DVOphthal MRCVS

John Robinson BDS (Lond)

Gairn Ross BVMS MRCVS and the 180 veterinary surgeons of the People's Dispensary for Sick Animals (PDSA)

David Scarff BVetMed CertSAD MRCVS

Jim Simpson SDA BVMS Mphil MRCVS

David Watson BVetMed MRCVS

David Williams MA VetMB CertVOphthal MRCVS

The Publishing Team: Sam, Viv, Jane, Alyson, Claire and Nina.

PUBLISHER'S ACKNOWLEDGEMENTS

Mitchell Beazley would like to thank the following organizations and people for their help with photography, illustrations and modelling:

Mr A Glue at Millbrooke Animal Centre (RSPCA), Chobham; Craig & Janet Irvine-Smith, Howard Taylor, Sue Holden, Liz McGauley and Anne Walton at Stonehenge Veterinary Hospital; Graham & Lesley Howlett & Rufus (our star cat model!); Vicky Gray; Alison, Mike & Grace Molan; Sue Oxley; Vera Lopez; Sarah Pollock: Nicola O'Connell; Tim Ridley; Rosie Hyde and Jane Burton.

PICTURE CREDITS

Animal Health Trust/Julia Freeman 21

Animal Graphics Ltd 60

University of Bristol/Dept of Clinical Veterinary Science/Dr John Innes 43 right

University of Bristol/Dept of Clinical Veterinary Science/Dr Paul Wooton 35 top

University of Bristol/Feline Advisory Bureau/Dr Andy Sparkes 37, 38, 67, 69, 73, 91

University of Edinburgh/Dept of Veterinary Clinical Studies/Dr Keith Thoday 48, 57 below

Jane Burton 1

Mark Evans 85, 113 left

In-Practice/BVA/Dr Keith Thoday 59

Journal of Small Animal Practice/R Harvey 57

Leo Animal Health 19 below, 20

Dr Ian Mason 50

Oxford Scientific Films/London Scientific Films 29 below left/John McCammon 81/Charles Tyler 125

Reed International Books Ltd/Jane Burton 2, 9 all, 15 below, 16 left, 17, 23, 41, 51, 55 below left, 56, 61, 62, 72, 79, 99 right, 99 left, 99 below, 101, 102 below, 103 top, 103 below left, 103 below right, 104 below right, 104 below left, 105, 106 left, 106 right, 107, 108, 110, 111 below, 111 top, 112, 113 right, 115, 116, 117, 118, 119 top, 119 below, 120, 121 below, 121 top, 123/Nigel Goodall 55 below right/Rosie Hyde – Stonehenge Veterinary Hospital 27, 31, 33, 71, 77, 89, 90, 92, 94, 95 top, 95 below, 96, 97/Tim Ridley 3, 6, 86, 87, 100 below right, 100 below left, 102 top centre, 102 top right, 102 top left, 124

Illustrations Stefan Chabluck 88, 89/Liz Gray 18, 28, 29, 43, 46, 54, 63, 65

Jacket photography Tim Ridley front, Rosie Hyde–Stonehenge Veterinary Hospital back below right, Tim Ridley below left, *Your Cat*/Lesley Deaves back flap

John Robinson BDS (Lond) 22, 24

Royal Veterinary College/Professor P. Bedford 13, 15 top left, 16 right

Solvay Duphar Veterinary Ltd 39

Mrs Alison (Couts) Speakman & Ms K Willoughby/In Practice 19 top, 25

Stonehenge Veterinary Hospital 45 top right, 45 top left, 46 left, 35 centre right, 35 top right, 35 below right

ZEFA Picture Library 7